HEALING WITH WATER

HEALING WITH WATER:

Special Applications and Uses of Water in Home Remedies for Everyday Ailments

Jeanne Keller

Illustrations by
Dorothea Sabine Koch

Parker Publishing Co., Inc.   **West Nyack, N. Y.**

Eighth Printing.....June, 1971

Library of Congress
Catalog Card Number: 68-31768

PRINTED IN THE UNITED STATES OF AMERICA
B & P

DEDICATION

TO MY GRANDCHILDREN

for a healthier and happier life

FOREWORD

During my entire practice as a Doctor of Medicine in Europe and my stay in the United States, I had a continuing interest toward natural healing methods. It was my particularly good opportunity to observe first-hand the remarkably effective results in Jeanne Keller's family which followed a system of applications of cold water under her direction as a healing and immunizing agent in a great variety of health situations.

I have never known anyone in her family, including her six grandchildren, to be in need of a doctor's attention. Bits and pieces of the effectiveness of cold water applications are generally known to practically all of us. Who does not remember when Mother placed a cold compress on a sore throat, or on a swelling caused by a cut or a physical blow?

However, a scant knowledge of such water applications is not enough for all benefits that may be possible in promoting health.

Jeanne Keller's book deals with a wide variety of health situations as she has handled them and I recommend her book for the readers' guidance in their own homes for securing glowing health. The book is easy to understand by the lay reader and cold water applications are described in good detail with illustrations.

Last, and by no means least, I also recommend the book because it shows how the various cold water methods can be used by anyone who wants to get a better measure of health without going to any extra expense.

Dr. Sabine Koch

INTRODUCTION

This book is the expression of a long and sincere desire to bring the knowledge of the various forms of water applications as means of healing to all those in need of help in securing better health. By familiarizing yourself with the various methods in this book and applying them for your various ailments you may enjoy vibrant health and the great happiness of uninterrupted well-being.

This book brings to you my experiences in curing a variety of ailments simply by the use of water in its various applications and also in connection with other natural healing agents.

In my belief that the acquaintance with a number of actual cases makes us wiser in carrying out the applications than the knowledge of abstract rules, I have itemized the procedures I followed in step-by-step action and in most cases a stated method is amplified by illustrations and detailed explanations and programs.

The book can also be used to advantage by those who wish to retain their health and the proper functioning of their body, or even to improve the functioning of a specific organ. They will find that water not only cleanses the body on the outside but also purifies it internally and creates a radiance of gloriously good health, strength and youth in inner feeling that anyone can't miss noticing about you.

After briefly telling you my first acquaintance with the benefits of cold water applications, the book proceeds immediately to specific cases and programs that were followed which include enough special applications to give a working knowledge of the water applications so that they may be safely applied by anyone who handles them conscientiously. The inclusion of a chapter on herbs and other natural healing agents at the end of the book adds to the useful benefits of the book for your maximum good health.

CONTENTS

11

List of Illustrations

HEALING WITH WATER

1

How the Secrets of Water Applications Help You Secure Glowing Health

Although medicine has made great strides in finding causes and cures for many ailments, the most sophisticated physician will generally admit that in spite of his vast technical knowledge, he knows comparatively little about the complexities of the human body in coping with attacks of bad health. Therefore, you will realize that we cannot afford to ignore any method which has been demonstrated in actual cases to be effective in reducing pain and suffering. Drugs have their place in an emergency and are a blessing at the right time and place, but I believe there is no drug known to science which does not exact a penalty for its prolonged use. "Side effects" of "miracle drugs" upon the body and mind may be serious, and possibly you may know of them by your own experience or by those of other persons.

I have applied cold water for numerous ailments and will tell you what I have learned. You and your family may be helped in similar cases to get relief from painful experiences and gain healing in due course.

What Water Application Will Do

I do not say that cold water cures you or heals your body. You know that even a physician cannot claim that he heals you; he cannot heal the smallest cut on your finger, but your body processes can do the healing. *All you and I, or a physician, can do, is to provide conditions or supplies that will assist, or induce, or help the body to heal itself.*

Neither do I claim that cold water is a cure-all. That would be quackery. All I know is that cold water has helped me and my family, as well as others, in many cases of illness to regain health and to keep vibrantly healthy throughout the years. For us water is the healing answer for many ailments, and it can also be the answer for you. You can easily convince yourself by starting with any simple application as outlined in this book.

My First Experience with Water Applications

My experience began when I was in Europe some years ago. I had a severe cold and because of it learned about the use of cold water as taught by Monsignor Sebastian Kneipp, who has become internationally famous for his "Kneipp water cures."

You will understand that I was rather skeptical at first, since I had always been told to keep warm when I had a cold. How could cold water help? I was inclined to believe that it would only make my cold worse. If contrary information had come from an ordinary layman's source, I should not have dared to put it to the test for my cold. However, since it originated from Monsignor Kneipp, I felt that I had good reason to believe it if I ever believed anything, because of his great number of healing successes using his water applications.

A Case of Double Pneumonia Healed

I also remembered at that time the only case I had ever known in which cold water had been applied, namely, my own father's case of double pneumonia when I was about fourteen years old. My father had been very ill for a number of days during which we children were not allowed to see him; neither could he have any other visitors, because he was delirious from a very high temperature. One day his delirium was so violent that he jumped out of bed. He screamed that his bed was on fire, and wanted to run out of the house. He could be retained only by force. Apparently our good house doctor, who lived next door and was always on call, could not do much for him. He had mentioned that the crisis was imminent and that he had very little hope for my father to pull through because of his weak heart.

In her great anguish my mother called one of my father's friends. He came over immediately and brought with him a physician who was new in town. I understood that this physician used certain natural methods in most illnesses and was connected with the Kneipp Sanatorium in the next town. What methods he used and how they were applied were not known to me at the time, but undoubtedly they were those described in the chapter on pneumonia in this book. I only remember that he sent for his daughter, apparently a trained nurse, who stayed with my father until all danger had passed. She called for buckets of cold water, pot cheese, pieces of linen, towels, etc. It was a time of great suspense and great heartache.

The next morning we heard to our relief and joy that my father's temperature had returned to normal. He was soaking wet from perspiration for a few hours, and we were told that this was a good sign. It meant that he was on the way to recovery. The spongings were continued and gradually reduced, while my father was getting his old strength back.

Water Healings Ever Available

It surprises me now that after this wonderful experience my mother did not attempt to learn more about the cold-water methods in order to apply them regularly for the family. She probably was of the opinion, as was I at the time, that these methods were merely applied in an emergency, and then only by a physician or trained nurse. How fortunate for you and me to know now that these water methods can be used safely and successfully by anyone at any time to obtain the blessings of living in vibrantly good health.

Cold Water Is the Answer in Coping With Ailments

My own experiences proved to me beyond all expectations and without a doubt that cold water is the answer for many ailments. Whenever we have used cold water as directed and planned, our colds and other illnesses simply disappeared into their native nothingness!

This knowledge has changed my whole life and can change yours also. I wish you could say with me that whereas I used to be rather worried about getting ill, now I am completely relaxed and happy in the assurance that I need not be afraid any more of most illnesses because I know what to do about them. I realize with a grateful heart that the water application is a glorious and valuable gift, and available to all sincerely seeking better health.

I did not start with the treatments for my cold until I arrived back in the United States and was in my own apartment, where I had all the conveniences and privacy. My husband did not approve at all of the cold-water applications. He simply could not believe in them, but he did not succeed in dissuading me. He finally said quite helplessly: "I hope you know what you are doing."

Although the favorable results I had should have convinced him, he did not want to use cold water for himself. In the beginning it took great persuasion to induce him to give it a try. Even after it had helped him once or twice he argued against it whenever I suggested using it. And when I reminded him of the successes he had had, he talked of "coincidence" or that the illness probably would have gotten better by itself. He also intimated that the cold-water applications most likely had helped me because I believed in them. My reply thereto and argument against it went about as follows:

"You don't have to believe in it at all. Even if you are convinced that it will not help, you will see that it does. Just give it a try. One need never fear that any cold-water application, if done correctly, could ever be bad for the body or any part of it. Any application directed toward a particular part is also at the same time beneficial to the whole body. Therefore, what chance do you take in trying?"

In the end he invariably agreed, with a certain amount of grumbling, to follow what I had proposed to do, and the results were always positive.

By the time our first daughter was born, he was so thoroughly convinced of the beneficial effects of cold water that he never questioned any application again and was absolutely confident that whatever form of cold-water application I used for the family was conducive to our health.

The Kneipp Sanatorium Experience

My husband's reluctance to use cold water surprised me somewhat because his own mother had been practically kept alive by cold-water treatments. However, she had not applied them so much at home, but instead had taken "the cure" at one of the Kneipp sanatoriums whenever she was in need of it. Therefore my husband was under the impression that there was much more to it then just the simple applications I used. Since his mother had never discussed the treatments in his presence, he was entirely ignorant and consequently had no idea how much good a simple cold-water application can do for one's health.

My husband remembers quite clearly that, before his mother turned to the Kneipp Sanatorium for help, when he was about ten years old, his father had a very serious and depressing talk with him, impressing on him that he should be good to his mother because she was very sick with lung hemorrhages, and, according to the doctor, would not live much longer. However, the cure at the Kneipp Sanatorium restored her to better health and strength, although she always looked very delicate. Once she was well again she kept up the cold-water applications only sporadically and finally dropped them entirely. When in later years the hemorrhages reappeared, she always turned again to cold water.

My husband is now over sixty, and his mother is still alive, and very much so. She runs the business her husband had left her very successfully and efficiently. Not only has she outlived her husband, but her two physicians, her three brothers and one sister as well.

Dramatic Benefits Secured with Water Applications

On one of my visits she told me herself that the Kneipp methods have kept her alive, not only applied for her lung hemorrhages but also for various other illnesses. She related to me one instance when, after a grave illness, her temperature had dropped to subnormal and her doctor was apparently at his wit's end to bring it back to normal. Although she was very weak and could not leave her bed, she wanted to take cold spongings. Everyone seemed to be against it in her condition, but she insisted on having a bucket with cold water put in front of her bed, with a small towel in it, and to be left alone. As weak as she was, she managed to sit on a chair in front of her bed, sponged herself off as well and as quickly as she could and got right back into bed again. (You will find a description of a full sponging in Chapter 2 under Case No. 1.)

She repeated this sponging routine every hour for a few hours. When the doctor came again the next day, her temperature was normal (and stayed normal). Her doctor knew that she often resorted to cold water. Therefore his first reaction was: "Don't tell me you used your foolish cold-water sponging again?" She affirmed this with a grin.

Healings through water applications have been thoroughly established. You have but to establish them for yourself in applying the simple programs of self-help in connection with the various health situations as set out in this book.

2

Getting Rid of a Cold
in the Head

Whenever a member of our family had a cold in the head, we used cold water either in the form of full spongings, as outlined in this chapter under Case No. 1, or full baths, as described under Case No. 2.

We find these methods a quick help at all times, invigorating, inexpensive but nevertheless very beneficial to all parts of the body without any negative effects. Since they have helped all of us they are sure also to help you and your family. If in the beginning you are not inclined to apply cold water to your whole body, then a cold upper sponging every hour for eight hours, or one every morning and evening (as described in Chapter 8, Case No. 1) would be a good start and definitely helpful for your cold. It can always be followed gradually by a full sponging or even a full bath whenever you are ready for it.

CASE No. 1

I felt very miserable, with a heavy, aching head and a stuffed nose. I could hardly look out of my eyes and had no taste for food at all. Following is the water application for this complaint:

FULL SPONGING:

One thorough sponging every hour for eight hours during the first day; one in the morning and one at night during the second day, for which the following "make-ready" is indicated:

PROVISIONS:

1. the bathroom and bedroom to be warm, or comfortable,
2. allow no draft due to open doors or windows,
3. two extra blankets on the bed.

SUPPLIES:

1. a good-sized facecloth.
2. a basin full of ice-cold water,
3. a bath or bed sheet (to reach from under the armpits to below the knees),
4. a bath towel.

PROCEDURE A:

1. I stepped quickly into the bathroom and undressed completely,
2. washed (sponged) myself as quickly as possible in even strokes, dipping the facecloth frequently and taking about one minute in all, in the following sequence:
   a. the chest and abdomen from the shoulders to the crotch,
   b. the entire back (see footnote *)
   c. the entire legs, front and back, including feet,
   d. the entire arms, front and back,
3. without drying myself, wrapped the bath sheet around me from under the armpits to the legs,

---

* I had practiced first with a dry facecloth to get a certain technique in flipping the cloth over my right shoulder with my left hand and pulling it with my right hand all the way down the right side of my back, then using the same procedure over my left shoulder with the hands reversed. Of course, it would have been much better if I had had someone wash my back.

      tucking one corner in on top, and draped the bath
      towel around my shoulders like a cape,
4. hurried back into bed and covered myself well,
      tucked in all around as much as possible, especially
      around the shoulders,
5. at one-hour intervals, repeated 1. to 4. seven times;
6. one hour after the last sponging got up and dressed
      warmly enough to feel comfortable.

If I had been too sick or too weak to get up, I would have arranged for someone to apply:

PROCEDURE B:

1. sponge me off in even strokes as follows:
    a. lying on my stomach, the entire back from the
       neck down to the hips,
    b. the back of the legs from the hips to the feet
       (without drying),
    c. lying on my back, the front of the legs and cover
       them up with the bedding without drying,
    d. chest and belly,
    e. arms,
2. cover me without drying up to my chin, well tucked
      in all around,
3. repeating 1. and 2. with one hour intervals seven
      times,
4. one hour after the last sponging, put on my pajamas
      to relax in bed.

If I had been too weak to get a whole sponging with cold water all at once, I should have arranged for someone to apply

PROCEDURE C:

(sponging split up into three sessions)
1. in the morning
    a. sponge the entire back in even strokes from the
       neck down to the thigh,
    b. without drying, cover me up well for one hour,
2. at noon
    a. sponge the chest and belly

      b. without drying, cover me up well for one hour,
  3. in the afternoon
      a. sponge the arms and legs (back and front)
      b. without drying, cover me up well for one hour
  4. repeating 1. to 3. every day for eight days.

Comments to Procedure A

After the first sponging I developed a very agreeable warmth. I was very relaxed, breathing deeply, and my head felt somewhat lighter. After a while the cold, however, took over again, and I was really looking forward to the second sponging because I had felt so good after the first one.

With each sponging I developed more warmth and even started to perspire after the third one. In spite of the perspiration I kept up the cold sponging (without drying myself before or after). I simply sponged the perspiration off, which did not stop it but increased it from hour to hour. My nose started to run freely without interruption accompanied by frequent sneezing, while my breathing became more and more easy through my nose. It seemed as if my cold was being washed out with great force all at once.

At the end of the day I felt very good, almost normal—except for my profusely running nose—my head was clear, breathing through my nose was normal, and I had a very good appetite.

After the second day my nose dried up gradually. It stopped running altogether after the third day. My head stayed clear and my appetite remained good. The cold sponging had taken care of my head cold entirely. It also had helped to loosen my cough somewhat. However, I felt that the latter required a more localized application which is described in Chapter 3.

In later years I found a short cut to get rid of a cold in the head which I describe in Case No. 2.

CASE No. 2

Whenever I became overworked on the job or at home, I came down with a cold. Following is an alternate program to the full sponging routine (Case No. 1):

FULL BATH:

One in the morning and one at night, for two days (see Chapter 10, 4).

Comments

One hour before retiring for the night I got ready for my cold bath as outlined under Insomnia, Chapter 10. While the tub was filling with cold water, I warmed up in bed. After having taken the cold bath and stayed wrapped up in bed for half an hour, I exchanged the bath sheet and bath towel for my pajamas, which I did as quickly as possible, covering up well again, and went to sleep.

In the morning I got up an hour earlier than usual. After having closed the windows I went right into the cold water which I had saved from the night before, and quickly back to bed. After half an hour I again exchanged the bath sheet and bath towel for my pajamas as quickly as possible and stayed in bed, well covered up, for another half hour, after which time I dressed and went about my usual daily routine.

I have found through the years that four of these cold full baths taken one in the morning and one at night for two days have cured not only my head colds but also those of my husband and our daughters, when they followed the cold-water routine.

However, usually after the first or second full bath it seems as if the cold were getting worse, because the nose starts running profusely, but the head gets clear right away and the breathing through the nostrils becomes easy. The headache and numbness disappear, appetite and sleeping return to normal, and for a while the cold is merely a local condition in the nose where all impurities seem to get washed out in a great house-cleaning.

After two days also the nose usually gets back to normal. Even in those cases where it kept running a day or two longer I did not continue the cold full baths beyond two days, and always was back to normal in a short time.

3

A Simple Way to Loosen
a Cough

Although my cough had improved somewhat with the cold spongings I had taken for the cold in my head, I still had coughing spells shortly after I went to bed and sometimes during the night. Therefore I decided to make a

COMPRESS ON THE CHEST:

Once a day, for as many days as needed, for which I arranged on a chair in front of my bed with the following:

SUPPLIES:

1. a bowl of cold water with about six ice cubes to keep it cold,
2. a good-sized facecloth, folded twice into four layers,
3. a face towel, folded double,
4. a small piece of thin rubber sheeting, larger, however than half the towel, to overlap all around, and followed the ensuing

PROCEDURE:

1. I went to bed for the night,
2. after having exposed my chest, dipped the facecloth into the water, wrung it out gently, not too dry,

neither dripping wet, and placed it (folded in four layers) on my upper chest, including part of the throat, to cover the area where I felt the irritation,

3. covered the compress with the folded dry towel in such a way that about an inch extended beyond the wet cloth on all sides so that no draft would get in,

4. placed over this the rubber sheeting extending about an inch beyond the towel all around, to prevent the bedding from getting wet,

5. pulled my blankets up high so that I was well covered up to my chin,

6. after about ten minutes checked the facecloth and found that it was getting warm, dipped it again into the cold water and proceeded as before,

7. continued checking twice more after fifteen minutes each, dipped the facecloth into the cold water and followed the same procedure,

8. after one hour removed all parts of the compress, making sure that I was not exposing my chest for too long, and covered myself well again up to the chin until I fell asleep.

Comments

After having applied the compress for about fifty minutes I stopped coughing, and went to sleep as soon as the hour was up and I had removed the compress. I slept very well that night without any coughing spells. However, I had one spell in the morning shortly before I got up. By then my cough was very loose and I was able to expectorate very easily and almost immediately.

I made another cold compress the following evening before going to sleep, the same as the night before, and my cough was gone the next day.

I have used this method for my whole family for more than thirty years with the usual quick results. A cough never lasted longer than two or three days if promptly attended to. If I had neglected any cough, more applications might have been necessary on successive days, but would have inevitably had the the same good end results.

4

Avoiding Adenoids

During my childhood I was rather plagued by adenoid trouble and repeated headaches. Breathing through my nose was rather difficult, until finally the adenoids had to be removed by operation when I was about ten years old. At that time we had also moved into another house with a large back yard, and I remember that I took every opportunity to walk barefoot in this back yard—even on the wet pavement—until I was about fifteen because it felt so good and I enjoyed it. Nobody had advised me to do so, but luckily nobody had kept me from doing it either. During those years the adenoids did not return, as they are usually inclined to do, and my headaches occurred only rarely and were much less severe.

I now realize that walking barefoot had brought the necessary improvement in my circulation and prevented the recurrence of the diseased adenoids. However, when I lived in New York City and did not have the benefit of a back yard where I could walk barefoot, the adenoids made themselves felt again. In order to prevent their condition from becoming severe, I used the following methods:

1. WALKING BAREFOOT:

all year whenever possible (for details see Chapter 13, Cases Nos. 1, 2, also comments)

2. NASAL RINSE WITH SCOURING RUSH:

(Latin: equisetum arvense—an herbal tea)
Five or six times daily for as many days as needed, for which
I made the following

PREPARATION:

1. I poured a cup of boiling water over one teaspoon
   of scouring rush,
2. letting it steep for five minutes,
3. strained it, and used the following

PROCEDURE:

1. I poured a small quantity of the warm herb tea into
   the palm of my hand
2. sniffed it up and drawing it slowly up into both
   nostrils,
3. repeated 1 and 2 four or five times at intervals of
   about an hour, mostly in the morning and evening.

Comments on 1. Walking Barefoot

My constantly walking barefoot whenever I have an opportunity
has done its part in preventing the recurrence of the adenoids. I
have never been troubled with them again.

In this connection I like to mention that my two daughters never
had the slightest sign of any adenoids because they walked barefoot from early childhood. When they were babies I never put
any socks or shoes on their feet and bought their first pair of
shoes only after they started walking and had to wear them on the
street. They never complained about cold feet. Even in cold
weather their feet were always warm.

Comments on 2. Nasal Rinse

Although this is a very mild tea, it actually "attacked" the
adenoids and seemed to dissolve them gradually without any pain
or discomfort, so that before long I could breath normally again
through my nose without the slightest effort.

5

Healing External Infections and Inflammations

Nothing seems to heal infections and inflammations so smoothly, painlessly, and completely as cold water. In its various applications, it may be as a spray, a cold compress, a compress with herbs, or a hayflower bath, either all of them in rotation or in any combination of them.

Spray Applications for Slight Infections

At the smallest sign of an infection I recommend spraying with cold water immediately, and that is usually the end of the infection. I am sure if you ever try it, you will have the same beneficial results. You may be wondering whether you should keep a wound dry, as is often advised, but then you would not have the healing power of water which will bring about much quicker results. Don't feel that water would do any harm, or be afraid if the wound after spraying turns red. The water can only do good if correctly and reasonably applied as provided generally in this book.

Aggravated Infections and Inflammations

The following three cases of a rather serious nature will give you a general idea what to do in case of an infection or inflammation.

CASE No. 1: INFECTION OF FINGER

I had developed an infection around the nail of my left ring finger. At first I did not pay any attention to it and later on did not have the time because of the preparations for my departure to heed urging to see a doctor. By that time I could not even wear a glove because of the swelling, and since my finger was hurting considerably, I had to protect it from any contact. When I was not even able to return to work, relief was obtained by the following program:

1. ARM SPRAY:

(for details and illustrations see also Chapter 24)
One every morning and afternoon, for as many days as needed, for which I arranged the following

SUPPLIES:

1. a rubber hose or hand spray (without the spray head) attached to the bathtub faucet,
2. a bath towel, and followed the ensuing

PROCEDURE:

1. Aside from removing my blouse, I stayed fully dressed and bent slightly over the bathtub,
2. sprayed my arm with the coldest water possible by holding the hose about three inches away at such an angle that the water covered the entire arm like a sheet (never in single streams or trickles);
   a. started at the fingertips, holding the hose for a few seconds right on the infected finger, and then proceeded slowly up the entire arm to the shoulder,
   b. held the hose for a moment on the shoulder, then proceeded slowly down again ending up at the fingertips,
   c. repeated a. and b. four more times,
3. without drying the arm, wrapped it at once in the dry bath towel and put a cardigan over my shoulder,

4. after half an hour removed the towel, wore my regular clothes and kept active and warm, leaving the finger uncovered as much as possible.

2. COLD COMPRESS

Once a day, for as many days as needed, for which I prepared the following

SUPPLIES:

1. a bowl of cold water with about six ice cubes to keep it cold,
2. a piece of kitchen towel (about a quarter of the towel), folded double to fit around the finger,
3. a face towel, and used the following

PROCEDURE:

1. I dipped the piece of toweling into the cold water, wrung it out gently (not too dry but neither dripping wet) and wrapped it around my finger,
2. covered the whole hand with the face towel to keep it warm,
3. after about ten minutes when the compress was getting warm, dipped the wet cloth again in the ice-cold water, proceeding as before,
4. repeated 3. every fifteen or twenty minutes for about one and a half hours,
5. removed the compress and wrapped my hand in a dry towel for another half hour to have the finger adjust to the normal temperature.

3. FINGER BATH

With hay flowers (an herbal tea), twice a day, morning and evening, for as many days as needed, for which I made the following

PREPARATION:

1. one teaspoon of hay flowers into one cup of boiling water,

2. letting it steep for about five minutes, and used the following

PROCEDURE:

1. I poured the herb tea into a glass and held my finger in it, moving it around freely, for about fifteen to twenty minutes,
2. wrapped the finger loosely in a dry bandage for half an hour,
3. left the finger uncovered as much as possible.

Comments on 1. Arm Spray

At first my arm felt really numb from the cold. It had become very red because the blood was rushing to the surface in order to fight off the cold produced by the water, thereby increasing circulation and accordingly also the healing process. After I had wrapped the bath towel around my arm, I felt an agreeable warmth filling my whole arm, with a pleasant tingling down to my fingertips.

If I had been unable to stand the cold water five times going up and down my arm, I should have started with two or three times and increased it with each spraying until I was able to take it five times.

Comments on 2. Compress

Right after the first application the strong pulsation in my finger diminished and the pain lessened considerably. It took the heat out of the infection, and after one and a half hours the pain was gone entirely.

Comments on 3. Finger Bath

The bath seemed to loosen the pus and wash it out at the same time. Upon light pressure the pus oozed out easily and the wound stayed open.

On the third day my finger was completely free of pus. Apparently no new pus had formed once I had started with the cold water spray and compress. There was no more pain, and the redness had almost completely disappeared. There was now a normal crust on the wound which came off in due time, and so did my fingernail, but a new one grew in perfect shape and consistency.

GENERAL

I was absolutely amazed at the quick healing of my finger, for which I have no medical explanation. I must have done the right thing to help the body heal itself, in the most magnificent manner.

I realize that the cold spongings I had taken for my head cold may have been at the same time instrumental in influencing the healing also of my finger, since they regulated the respiration and blood circulation of my entire body.

If I had not experienced such a fast healing of my finger I should have continued with the arm sprays each morning and evening and also with the compresses and finger baths until I had achieved complete healing.

CASE No. 2: EYE INFLAMMATION

I awoke one morning and could not open my right eye because the eyelids were stuck together. After I had washed my face I found that my eye was infected and inflamed, apparently resulting from a severe cold.

Following is the program to cope with this delicate situation:

1. EYE COMPRESS:

One in the morning and one at night for as many days as necessary for which I assembled the following

SUPPLIES:

1. a small handkerchief, folded twice (into four layers),
2. a small bowl with cold water (containing four ice cubes)
3. a hand towel, and followed this

PROCEDURE:

1. I dipped the folded handkerchief into the cold water and wrung it out lightly, not too dry, but neither dripping wet, and placed it on the eye,

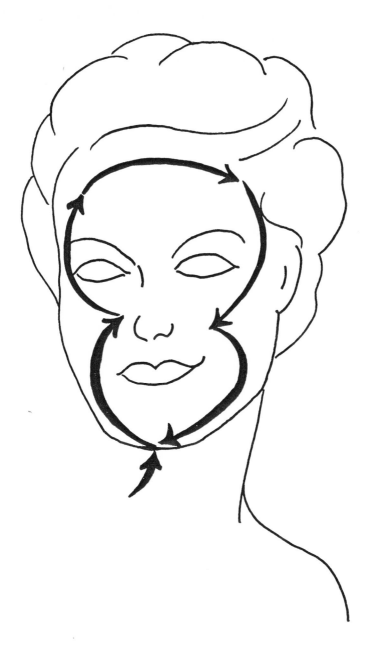

Figure 1: Face Spray—Arrows show directions of water spray.

2. covered it with the dry hand towel, making sure that no draft could enter,

3. whenever the handkerchief got warm, dipped it again and repeated in the same manner, always making sure that the handkerchief remained cool,

4. after an hour dried the eye, but kept it covered with a dry handkerchief for about half an hour to get it adjusted to the room temperature.

2. FACE SPRAY:

(Figure No. 1 on page 39 shows you the direction of the water spray.)
Early in the morning, four or five times each week, for which I arranged the following

SUPPLIES:

1. a rubber hose (or hand spray without the spray head) attached to the bathtub faucet,

2. a bathing cap,

3. a dry face towel, and followed this

PROCEDURE:

1. I put on my bathing cap and bent my face over the bathtub,

2. sprayed my face with the coldest possible water, holding the hose about three inches away, and starting at the right side of my face, going around in a circle and holding the hose an extra second or two on each eye,

3. repeated as outlined under 2, four or five times,

4. patted my face dry.

Comments on 1. Cold Compress

As soon as I put the cold compress on my eye the pain diminished. It had a cooling and very soothing effect. At the end of the first hour the inflammation had already been reduced, and in the evening the eye felt and looked much better. Nevertheless I applied the compress again for an hour. However, the following morning

I applied it for half an hour only. By that time my eye was almost normal. In the evening I repeated the compress again for half an hour, and the next morning there was no more sign of an inflammation and I discontinued the compresses.

Comments on 2. Face Spray

The third day I started taking the face sprays in order to strengthen my eyes and prevent further inflammations and infections. When I found that this spray was very refreshing and also beneficial to my skin and the texture of my face, I continued taking the face spray regularly, and still do.

CASE No. 3: STY ON THE EYE

My younger daughter one day developed a sty on her left eye. At first we did not pay much attention to it and expected it to go away by itself, as one had before. However, it soon became painful. The following water application method was used with excellent results.

COMPRESS ON EYE:

One hour in the morning and one at night, daily for 3 days (for details see Case No. 2, also Comments). If we had not had quick results we should have applied a

POT-CHEESE PLASTER:

One hour in the morning and one at night, daily for three days (for details see Chapter 19, Case No. 1), or a

SCOURING-RUSH COMPRESS:

One hour in the morning and one at night, daily for three days (for details and procedure see Case No. 2), with the following

PREPARATION:

1. two cups of boiling water poured over one tablespoonful of scouring rush (an herb tea),
2. letting steep for ten minutes,

3. after straining, handkerchief (folded into four layers) dipped into tea, wrung out lightly and applied as given under Case No. 2.

Comments on Compress on Eye

It was amazing how quickly the cold-water compress took the pain out of the sty, and after one hour the size was reduced considerably. The following morning there was no more pus in the sty. It looked as if it had drained out by itself. There was just a red spot left, and at the end of three days there was no more sign of any sty. The eye just felt and looked completely normal.

6

Relieving Tonsillitis

Tonsillitis, with the very disagreeable symptoms of weariness, high temperature, lack of appetite, difficulty in swallowing even liquids, can be made to yield to the water-cure method. In my experience, I found the following program very effective:

1. THROAT WRAPPING:

(see Figure 2 for correct application)
One wrapping daily, for as many days as needed, for which I arranged on a chair in front of my bed the following

SUPPLIES:

1. a bowl of cold water with about six ice cubes to keep it cold (never applying the ice cubes directly to my body, which would be too drastic),
2. a small kitchen towel, folded twice lengthwise to fit around my neck,
3. a small, thin bath towel, also folded twice lengthwise but wide enough to overlap the kitchen towel about an inch on both sides,
4. a small piece of rubber sheeting, wide enough to overlap the bath towel on both sides, and followed this

43

PROCEDURE:

1. I placed the rubber sheeting underneath my neck,
2. placed the folded bathtowel on top of the rubber sheeting,
3. dipped the folded kitchen towel into the water, wrung it out gently, neither dripping wet nor too dry, and wound it around my neck,
4. wrapped the folded bathtowel around the wet towel, not too tightly, but fitting closely,
5. wrapped the rubber sheeting around the bath towel, making certain that no air could come in, either at the top or the bottom,
6. pulled my blankets up high in order to be well covered up to my chin,
7. after about ten minutes checked the kitchen towel, which was getting warm, and dipped it again in the cold water, proceeding as before,
8. repeated the procedure outlined under 7. about every fifteen to twenty minutes,
9. after one and a half hours removed the entire compress and stayed in bed covered up to my chin for another half hour.

2. ALUM-WATER GARGLE:

Once every five minutes during first hour, once every fifteen minutes during second hour, thereafter once morning and evening for three days, with the following

PREPARATION:

One half teaspoon of powdered alum in a glass of cold water, stirred well until dissolved,

PROCEDURE:

Gargle each time once thoroughly and repeat as indicated before.

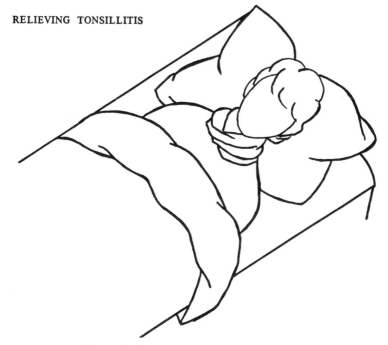

Figure 2: Throat Wrapping in proper position.

3. HALF BATH:

(see Figure 3 following for correct application)
One a day, for two days, thereafter one a week for prevention,
for which I made the following

PROVISIONS:

1. the bedroom and bathroom sufficiently warm,
2. no draft from any window or door,
3. sufficient blankets on my bed, and prepared the
   following

SUPPLIES:

1. the tub filled with enough very cold water to cover
   my hips,
2. a bath sheet placed in readiness,
3. a cardigan worn over my pajama top, and followed
   this

PROCEDURE:

1. I went to bed for about twenty minutes to get warm and also have the bed warm for my return after the cold bath,
2. stepped quickly into the bathroom,
3. rolled up my pajama top and cardigan, and tied them firmly in a knot (to keep them from getting wet), removing my pajama pants,
4. stepped into the tub and sat down immediately but slowly (see sketch),
5. counted ten seconds thus: "one and twenty, two and twenty, etc., to thirty (which gave me the correct timing for each second),
6. stepped out of the tub at the count of thirty, shaking the water off somewhat,
7. without drying myself, wrapped the bath sheet firmly around my hips, tucking the corner in at the waist,
8. rolled the cardigan and pajama top down and hurried back to bed, covering up well and tucked in especially around my hips,
9. after an hour dressed fully and went about my usual activities.

Comments on 1. Throat Wrapping

The first wrapping felt very soothing and seemed to take the heat out of my throat. The throbbing diminished considerably and I felt a great relief. I made sure to check after the first ten minutes so that the compress (wrapping) would not get warm because a warm compress would only make the condition worse. With each new dipping the relief increased and the swallowing became easier. However, a really marked improvement was felt only the next day.

Comments on 2. Alum-Water Gargle

Once the cold compress (wrapping) had taken the heat and pressure out of my throat, the gargling cleansed from the inside and contributed to the healing. After each gargling I was able to ex-

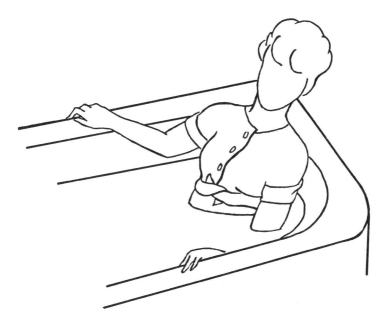

Figure 3: Half Bath showing proper position.

pectorate more and more easily; a great quantity of mucus was loosened and discharged, and the soreness diminished gradually.

Comments on 3. Half Bath

I felt that the half bath was drawing the pressure away from my throat and normalizing the blood circulation, thereby assisting the body additionally in the healing of my throat.

Before getting out of bed for the half bath, I made it clear to myself that as little time as possible should be lost, once I had gotten out of bed, until I stepped into the tub. Therefore once I had made up my mind to go through with it, I did not hesitate in front of the tub, knowing that it is important for the body to remain warm.

I must admit that it is still not easy for me, after all these years of taking a half bath, to step into the tub and sit down in the cold water, but I have learned that it is much easier to do it immediately than to stand in front of the tub and hesitate, and once I am sitting down, the cold feeling passes quickly and it seems just as easy to stay in the cold water ten seconds as a few seconds.

If I had been too weak to take a half bath, I should have started with a knee spray (see Chapter 11, 2) for two or three days and then continue with a half bath of two or three seconds, gradually increasing it each day to ten seconds.

The favorable reaction after the half bath was quite remarkable. I felt calm and relaxed. My breathing was slow and deep. The lower part of my body felt very warm as soon as I got into bed. The blood circulation seemed to be rather lively, but my pulse was steady. I felt a tingling all through my body, even into the tips of my fingers.

The next day my throat was much better, and after the second day I had only a trace of throat discomfort, which disappeared very soon. I was happy that through these applications the tonsillitis was cured in two days; formerly such a cure had taken at least two weeks.

Because of the great benefits I derived from the half bath, I have taken one each week whenever possible ever since, and I have never had another case of tonsillitis for more than thirty-five years.

GENERAL

Sometimes the thought entered my mind that I might have outgrown the tendency for tonsillitis, but during the fall of 1966 I was again convinced that the cold half baths had prevented it. At that time we had spent our vacation in our ski cabin in the White Mountains, where we did not have any modern facilities. For three weeks I had not been able to take any half baths. The weather was colder than expected and we did not have enough warm clothing with us. But this did not keep us from spending most of our time outside and really roughing it, with the result that I got not only tonsillitis, but also laryngitis. However, I did not feel sick, but went about my usual activities. These conditions remained in my throat until we returned home, where I immediately took up the cold half baths again, and the next day my voice had returned and I could swallow easily again.

7

Cleaning and Healing Boils

If you ever had a boil, then you know how painful and disturbing they can be, and if you should happen to have a boil just now, then you may want to try the applications given under cases Nos. 1 and 2 of this chapter and experience for yourself how wonderfully it can be healed. However, if you or your child should suffer from many boils, the following may guide you in your applications:

When my brother was about one year old, he had a number of boils on various parts of his body. Apparently our family doctor could not do much for him, and the following steps were taken:

My mother bathed my brother for a week every morning in lukewarm hay flower water for about fifteen minutes, with the result that the pus came oozing out of the boils very easily and the boils healed within a short time. She took about three cups of hay flowers, steeped them in boiling water and added them to the bath water. It would have also been advisable for my mother to give my brother a full bath every afternoon for a week (for details check in Chapter 19, 2); then he would have gotten his strength back much more quickly. Also, a short wrapping would have been very beneficial (for details see Chapter 8, No. 1, 5).

CASE No. 1: BOIL ON THIGH

My husband told me of a very annoying boil he had on his thigh and because of which he could only sit on one side. The following program was used with excellent results:

1. HIP SPRAY:

(see Figures 4 and 5 on next pages for correct application)
One a day, for seven days, for which he should make the following

PROVISIONS:

1. the bedroom and bathroom to be warm,
2. no draft anywhere because of open doors or windows,
3. 2 extra blankets on his bed, and arrange for the following

SUPPLIES:

1. a rubber hose (or handspray without the spray head) attached to the bathtub faucet,
2. a large bath sheet in readiness,
3. a sweater over his pajama top, thereafter follow this

PROCEDURE:

1. go to bed for about twenty minutes or do exercises to get warm,
2. after having stepped into the bathroom, roll up the pajama top and sweater sufficiently to prevent them from getting wet at the waist,
3. remove the bottom part of the pajamas and step quickly into the empty bathtub,
4. spray with the coldest possible water in a very accurate manner (see sketch), holding the hose about three inches away in such a fashion that the water covers the entire leg like a sheet (not running in trickles),
   a. start at the heel of your right foot at No. 1

proceed the first time quickly up your leg until you have reached the upper part of your hip, No. 2 (keeping the hose itself away from the spine), going down quickly again until you have reached the heel, No. 1,

b. repeat the same course on the back of your left leg, from No. 3 to No. 4 and back,

c. repeat a. and b. very slowly two or three times more, i.e., right, left, right, left, holding the hose each time a few seconds on the boil,

d. turn around and start at the toes of your right leg, No. 1, going quickly up to your waist, No. 2, and then quickly down again, to No. 1,

e. repeat the same course on the front of your left leg, from No. 3 to No. 4 and back,

f. repeat d. and e. very slowly twice or three times, right left, right left,

5. without drying yourself, wrap the bath sheet tightly around your hips, tucking the outside corner in at the waist,

6. roll down your pajama top and sweater,

7. literally run into bed and cover up well, tucked in especially around the hips,

8. after half an hour remove the bath sheet, but remain in bed for altogether an hour.

2. COMPRESS ON BOIL:

One a day, for as many days as needed (see COUGH, Chapter 3). (The compress may not be necessary if the hip spray yields prompt results.)

Comments on 1. Hip Spray

I had added to my instructions that if he was unable to stand the cold spray three or four times going up and down each leg, back and front, then we should start first with once or twice and increase the following day to 3 or 4 times. I had also cautioned him not to lose too much time between getting undressed, taking the cold spray, and getting back into bed.

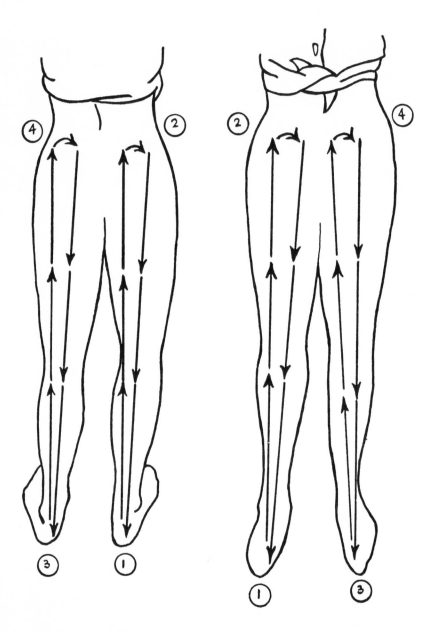

Figure 4: Hip Spray—Arrows indicate direction of water spray, front and back of body.

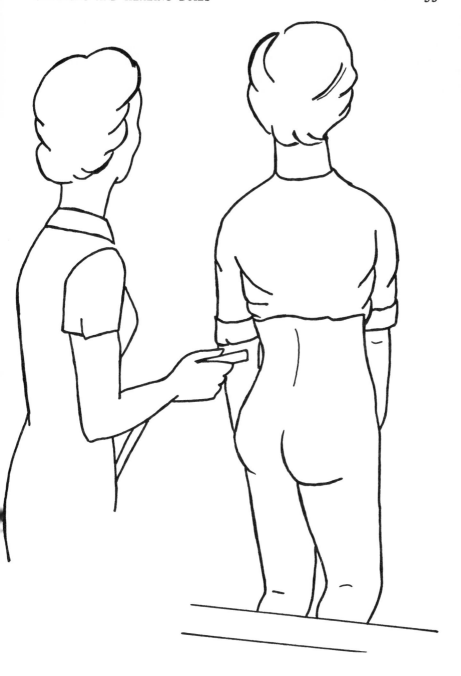

Figure 5: General technique in applying Hip Spray by another person.

The pressure and pain diminished immediately. We repeated the spraying on three successive days with the result that the boil softened gradually and soon disappeared entirely. He was never troubled again with this condition.

CASE No. 2: BOIL UNDER ARMPIT

I had developed a boil under my right arm. This was brought about by carelessness. I had cut myself while shaving and had played tennis soon afterward. The cut was rather irritating but I did not pay any attention to it, expecting it to take a while to heal. However, it became very painful after a few days, and one morning I realized that I had a good-sized and ugly boil under my arm. Well-meaning friends urged me to see a doctor immediately to have it cut open. They were horrified that I intended to treat it myself. I started immediately with

1. ARM SPRAY:

One in the morning and one at night, for two days, thereafter one in the morning as many days as needed (For details see Chapter 24).

2. PLASTER OF FENUGREEK SEED:

(Latin: Trigonella foenumgraecum)
One in the morning and one at night for two days, thereafter one in the evening for as many days as needed, for which I arranged the following

SUPPLIES:

1. to a tablespoonful of fenugreek seed in powder form I added gradually sufficient boiling water to make a thick paste, stirring it for about two minutes,
2. a small piece of cotton material about three inches square, big enough to cover the boil, with about an inch overlap all around,
3. four layers of gauze about three inches square,
4. two strips of tape about six inches long, and followed this

PROCEDURE:

1. I placed the two tapes on a table about one inch apart, adhesive side up, and placed the gauze on top with the tape extending one and a half inches on each side,

2. spread the paste on the piece of cotton material with a knife (just like spreading peanut butter) about half an inch thick, in a circle the size of the boil, and placed it on top of the gauze, with the paste side up,

3. attached the assembled plaster under my armpit so that it centered on the boil, pressing the ends of the tape down firmly on both sides,

4. removed the plaster only at night (or in the morning) shortly before I was ready to apply the next one,

5. after the wound was healed, removed the plaster and put a piece of dry gauze loosely in its place for about two days.

Comments on 1. Arm Spray

See INFECTION OF FINGER, Chapter 5, Case No. 1.

Comments on 2. Plaster of Fenugreek Seed

When I first applied the plaster it was very soothing and reduced the pain immediately. I was amazed that it drew out the pus absolutely painlessly and very thoroughly. Although I did nothing else to wash out or clean the wound, whenever I changed the plaster, it looked clean and dry, but remained open until all the pus had been drawn out. Only after the wound had no more yellow spots and just looked red and raw, did it start to heal.

The plaster always came off very easily. It never stuck to the wound. After a few days the wound looked very neat and dry, and soon it was completely healed.

I was able to go to work every day and experienced no discomfort. Soon afterward I played tennis again without any bad effects. I also continued shaving and never had another boil.

8

Strengthening and Improving Bladder and Kidneys

It seems strange that although water is often the cause of a bladder or kidney ailment, it is also its wonderful cure if properly applied. If you use cold water regularly, your bladder and kidneys will be strengthened and will not be so easily susceptible to colds and inflammations. Of course, it is always good to use reasonable precautions. For instance, if you get chills in a wet bathing suit on the beach, then you should dress immediately and exercise to get warm. There is a great difference between having a wet wrapping on your body while being well covered in bed, and having a wet bathing suit on while being exposed to the air. In the first instance the wrapping works beneficially on your body (see Chapter 40), while in the second case the wetness is likely to bring on a cold.

This chapter has the applications for four cases of bladder and and kidney troubles which may be of help to you in case of need.

CASE No. 1: BLADDER TROUBLE

Ever since my teens I have had bladder trouble at the slightest provocation with all its disagreeable symptoms, although I dressed particularly warmly during the winter, so much so that my hip measurements (over my skirt) increased considerably. But the

56

warmer I dressed the more susceptible I became. I remember that it felt particularly good to sit on a warm radiator. Even after having gone to the beach one hot summer day, I experienced great pain and discomfort during the night. I never consulted a physician because I considered it a mere cold. However, since I had learned about cold-water treatments and their strengthening effects, I applied some of them during the summer of 1934 as follows:

1. HIP SPRAY:

On Monday, Wednesday and Friday (for one week only), (see BOIL ON THIGH, Chapter 7, Case No. 1.)

2. HALF BATH:

On Tuesday, Thursday and Saturday of first week, on Mondays and Thursday during ensuing six weeks, thereafter one each week, (see TONSILLITIS, Chapter 6)

3. UPPER SPONGING:

Every morning for one week only, for which I made the following

PROVISIONS:

1. the bedroom and bathroom were warm,
2. there was no draft,
3. there were two extra blankets on my bed, and arranged for the following

SUPPLIES:

1. a basin full of the coldest water possible,
2. a good-sized facecloth,
3. a bath towel to tuck in around my waist during sponging,
4. a bath towel to wrap around my shoulders afterwards.

Since I felt cold, I went back to bed for a while to get comfortably warm. Then I followed this

PROCEDURE:

1. I tucked one bath towel around my waist to prevent my pajama pants from getting wet and to keep the lower part of my body warm,
2. removed my pajama top,
3. washed the upper part of my body in even strokes as quickly as possible, taking less than a minute, and dipping the facecloth frequently, in the following sequence:
   a. the back from the shoulders to the waist (see footnote on page 26),
   b. the front from the shoulders to the waist,
   c. underneath the right arm, going up from the fingertips to the shoulder, then down again on the outside of arm,
   d. the left arm in the same way,
5. without drying myself, put the dry bath towel around my shoulders like a cape and discarded the towel from the waist,
6. went to bed as fast as possible, pulling the covers up to my chin and tucking them in (from underneath) under my shoulders and arms, to eliminate any draft,
7. after half an hour got up and dressed, but kept active for another half hour in the house before going out.

4. HAY-FLOWER COMPRESS ON ABDOMEN:

One only (on Saturday of first week) for which I arranged, in front of my bed, the following

SUPPLIES:

1. to one and a half heaping tablespoons of hay flower in a large bowl, I added one and a half quarts of boiling water, letting the mixture steep for about ten minutes,
2. two kitchen towels, one third folded over at the narrow ends so that each towel had three layers,

together six layers, large enough to cover the abdomen,
(If I had felt very weak, I should have used only one
kitchen towel.)
3. a bath towel folded in the same manner,
4. a piece of thin rubber sheeting, large enough to
overlap the folded bath towel by about an inch on
all sides, and followed this

PROCEDURE:

1. I went to bed, rolled down the pajama pants to
uncover the abdomen,
2. dipped the kitchen towels together into the warm,
unstrained hay-flower solution, wrung them out
carefully (not too dry, but not dripping wet) and
put them on my abdomen, as low as possible, making
them cling to each side,
3. covered the kitchen towels with the bath towel which
extended about one inch beyond the kitchen towels
on all sides,
4. placed the rubber sheeting over the bath towel,
overlapping an inch on all sides,
5. covered up warmly with the regular bedding,
6. after forty-five minutes dipped the kitchen towels
again and applied as before, this time cold,
7. after another forty-five minutes removed the entire
compress and, without drying, covered up well for
about another half hour to feel warm and comfortable, getting up thereafter and going about my work.

5. SHORT WRAPPING:

One only (on Sunday of the first week)
Chapter 40 will guide you in its applications and give you a
complete outline, including the following figures:
Figure 28: showing you the correct application made with
the assistance of another person,
Figure 29: suggesting a way of applying the short wrapping
unaided, i.e., how it can be self-applied.

In this particular case I arranged in front of my bed the following

SUPPLIES:

1. to four heaping tablespoons of hay flowers in a large bowl I added four quarts of boiling water, letting it steep for about ten minutes,
2. a bedsheet 108″ long, folded twice (once in the length and once in the width), resulting in four layers and to reach from under the armpits almost down to the knees,
3. a woolen blanket folded double,
4. thin rubber sheeting to extend about an inch at the top and bottom of the folded blanket, and followed this

PROCEDURE:

1. I lined the bed with the rubber sheeting,
2. placed the folded blanket on the rubber sheet,
3. dipped the folded bedsheet into the warm, unstrained herb tea, wrung it out carefully (not too dry, but not dripping wet) and spread it on the blanket, with the latter extending about an inch on the top and the bottom.
4. placed myself—completely undressed—on the wet sheet in such a way that the upper edge reached to my armpits,
5. folded the sides of the wet sheet over myself, to cling closely to my body, first the one side and then the other, overlapping each other and closing well on top and bottom so that no air could come in,
6. folded the sides of the blanket over in the same manner, closing well on the top and the bottom, but not too tight,
7. put my pajama top and a cardigan over my arms, backside in front and tucked in on the sides, so that I could keep my arms out,
8. covered up warmly with the regular bed covers up

to my armpits and tucked in under my shoulder blades,

9. dipped the sheet again after forty-five minutes, this time in the cold hay-flower solution, by pulling the wet sheet from under me while still under the bed covers, dipping it with only one arm exposed, then wringing it out with both hands while lying on my stomach, and lifting myself slightly on my knees while spreading the wet sheet on the bed, with the bed covers still over my back all the time, then turning on my back again and repeating 4. to 8.

10. removed the entire wrapping after another forty-five minutes, put on my pajamas and covered up well in bed for about forty minutes to feel comfortably warm, getting up thereafter and going about my work.

Comments on 1. Hip Spray

When I had covered up in bed after the hip spray, I felt immediately an inner warmth circulating through my body and a tingling sensation all over my skin, even as far out as my fingertips, although I had not wet my arms. I was completely relaxed and breathing very deeply. I really felt good all over.

Comments on 2. Half Bath

I had similar sensations as after the hip spray. (See also under TONSILLITIS, Chapter 6)

Comments on 3. Upper Sponging

Before getting out of bed for the upper sponging I made it clear to myself that as little time as possible should be lost once I had gotten out of bed until I stepped back into bed. Therefore once I had made up my mind to go through with it, I did not hesitate in front of the sink, but started washing immediately so that my body remained warm.

After I had finished sponging and was back in bed, the skin of my upper body felt very warm and alive, as if the blood circulation was increased and brought into a good balance with the circulation of my entire body, complementing the hip spray from the night before. Again my breathing was deep and I was relaxed. When I got up half an hour later I felt very much alive.

Comments on 4. Hay-Flower Compress

When I applied the compress on my abdomen, it felt very warm. However, soon the compress cooled off and for a short while it felt a little cold, clammy and not very pleasant on my abdomen. But this state passed rather quickly and a very comfortable warmth developed. I was so much relaxed that I fell asleep for about half an hour. At the end of the compress my abdomen felt soft and relaxed.

A plain cold-water compress on the abdomen has helped me greatly in the case of tonsillitis. It also draws the blood away from the heart and after a short while an overactive heart starts beating normally and quietly.

Comments on 5. Short Wrapping

When I applied the short wrapping it also felt warm at first, but after it cooled off I felt uncomfortable and clammy for about two minutes, after which the wrapping became increasingly warmer, and soon I was completely relaxed and fell asleep for a while.

When I repeated the wrapping and applied it cold, I was chilled just for a moment, but that passed quickly and a comfortable warmth developed. Again I fell asleep because I was so perfectly relaxed.

After I had removed the entire wrapping, I felt light and clean, as if a lot of impurities had been drawn out of my body.

Of course, it would have been preferable if I had had help with the wrappings, especially the second one, for I took great pains in getting it ready without exposing myself unduly and without losing too much time. I was very much aware of the fact that the more thoroughly and carefully it was done, the more beneficial it would be.

If I had been weak or very old with a poor blood circulation, I should have applied the second wrapping warm also and should have used only half a bedsheet folded into two layers only.

I found this wrapping the most beneficial of all the applications and understand that if healthy people take it once a week or once a month, a lot of sickness can be prevented. It it supposed to purify the kidneys and liver, and to be beneficial for the intestines, stomach, heart, lungs, and even head and throat.

GENERAL

I was amazed that after two days I noted already an improvement in my bladder condition, and around the fourth and fifth day I was already inclined to stop the applications. However, I was wise enough to realize that in order to cure the condition once and for all I had to go through the entire program, which I managed without missing a single day at work.

At the end of the first week I had no more symptoms whatsoever; I just felt great. However, it seemed that I needed a little more sleep than usual. But it was wonderful to sleep so soundly, and my appetite was tremendous, without increasing my weight. In fact, I lost a few pounds during that time. All urinary functions were absolutely normal thereafter.

In order to keep healthy I continued taking a half bath once a week, balanced with arm sprays and an occasional upper sponging.

For the past many years my bladder and kidneys have functioned normally, even during pregnancy. I never needed heavy underwear again, but have been, and still am, wearing the same light underwear all year around.

If the trouble had recurred I simply should have given myself the same applications again, either in part or all of them, until perfect results had been obtained.

CASE No. 2: KIDNEY TROUBLE

While I was staying alone in our house I had a friend living with me to keep me company. The first evening, before she retired she asked me for two extra pillows to keep her kidneys warm because they were very sensitive and often caused her pain. As you will have read under Case No. 1, I used various cold water applications in order to improve my weak bladder. My friend was quite impressed and urged me to suggest to her what she could do to strengthen her kidneys. Of course, I could tell her only what I should do in her case, namely start with light applications and follow them later with stronger ones in this manner:

1. FULL SPONGING:

One daily during first week, one every other day during second week (see Chapter 2, Case No. 1, also Comments).

2. KNEE SPRAY:

One daily during first week, one every other day regularly thereafter (see Chapter 11, 2, also Comments).

3. SHORT WRAPPING:

One every other day during first week, twice a week during second and third week (see Chapter 40, also Figures 28 and 29).

4. HIP SPRAY:

One every other day during second and third week, once a week regularly thereafter (see Chapter 7, Case No. 1, also Comments).

5. BACK SPRAY:

One every other day during second and third week in alternation with hip spray, twice during third week (see Chapter 12, 3, also Comments).

Comments on 4. Hip Spray

My friend felt that she was strong enough to start immediately with the hip spray and asked me to apply it for her because she did not have the courage to do it herself. However, she had enough will power to hold still while I gave her a short spray for the first time. After she was warmly wrapped up in bed she exclaimed how wonderful it felt, how invigorating and at the same time relaxing. Because she felt so good now, she was sorry that she did not hold out for three repetitions of the spray. However, from then on she was willing to "endure" the full spray.

At the end of the second week there was a marked improvement in her condition; she had no more pain, her kidneys felt comfortable all through the day and night so that the two extra pillows during the night were no longer necessary, and she also dispensed with some of the extra underwear during the day. All in all, she was very happy about the good results.

In the fall of that year I moved to Boston and stayed in contact with her by mail. After a few years she wrote me that her old ailment was bothering her again, but she did not have the will power to apply the hip sprays herself. She expressed the wish that there would be someone "after her with a stick."

CASE No. 3: BED-WETTING

If bed-wetting is a problem for a child the following program is beneficial in controlling this condition:

1. WALK IN COLD WATER:

Twice daily, for two weeks, once daily thereafter for four weeks (see Chapter 13, Case No. 1, also Comments).

2. HALF BATH:

Three times a week, during third and fourth week (see Chapter 6, Case No. 3, also Comments).

3A. UPPER SPONGINGS:

Three times a week, during third and fourth week (see this chapter, Case No. 1, also Comments).
or

3B. UPPER SPRAY:

Once a week during third and fourth week (see Chapter 11, 1, also Comments).

4. HERB TEA MIXTURE:

One cup daily, taken one-third morning, noon, and night, for four weeks.

PREPARATION:

1. Pour one cupful of boiling water over one-half teaspoonful of sage leaves (cut) and one-half teaspoonful of scouring rush,
2. cover and let steep for five to ten minutes.

Comments on 1. Walk in Cold Water

Whenever my children walked in cold water during the day, they did not go to bed to get warm, but put on their socks and shoes immediately, without drying their legs and feet, and kept active by walking or running until they felt warm and dry, which was done in the house during cold weather and outside during the warm season.

GENERAL

If you put these methods to the test, you may have good results already within a few days. However, the older the child the longer it may take. Altogether these applications will bring the entire system into good functioning, and the child will feel better and stronger than he ever did.

CASE No. 4: BLADDER INFECTION

One day my daughter had developed a bladder infection which stayed with her for quite a while and was often rather painful, with blood discharge. The following water applications were used with satisfying results:

1. LOCAL STEAMBATH:

(see Figure 6 following for correct application)
One the first day, one the second day if needed with the following

PREPARATIONS:

1. two heaping tablespoonfuls of scouring rush to two quarts of boiling water,

2. a commode or pail next to the bed
3. a blanket in readiness, and this

PROCEDURE:

1. Pour hot herb tea into commode (or pail)
2. undress fully except for pajama top and sweater,
3. sit on commode or pail so that the steam rises against your body for about twenty to thirty minutes, with blanket draped around the lower part of your body,
4. after completion of steam bath, go to bed immediately without drying yourself, covering up with the regular bedding, not too heavy, so that the perspiration diminishes gradually,
5. after about an hour, when perspiration has stopped, take a

2. FULL SPONGING:

(for details see Chapter 2, Case No. 1) followed at night with

3. COMPRESS ON ABDOMEN:

One the first day, one the second day if needed, with scouring rush, hay flowers, or half vinegar and water (for details see Chapter 8, Case No. 1).

4. SCOURING RUSH TEA:

One swallow at a time every ten or fifteen minutes less often the next day(s) with the following

PREPARATION:

1. one flat teaspoonful to a cup of boiling water,
2. letting it steep for about 10 minutes and strain, these procedures to be followed by

5. HIP SPRAY,
6. HALF BATH,
7. UPPER SPONGING:

(for details see Chapter 8, Case Nos. 1, 2, 3)

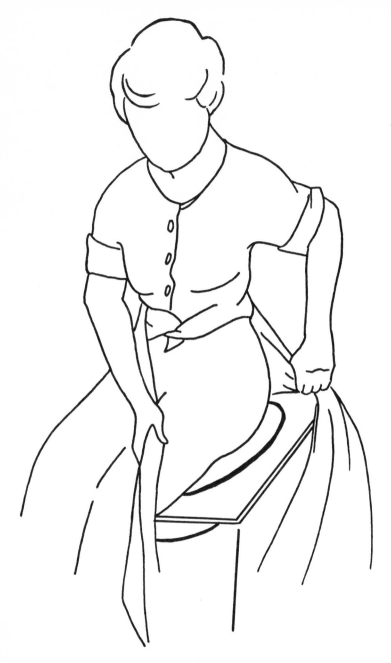

Figure 6: Positioning for localized Steam Bath.

Comments on 1. Local Steambath

It is unbelievable how a simple method as this local steambath can take care of an extremely disagreeable and often painful condition in such a short time. I can only say that trying and experiencing is believing. I know from my own experience that even if one has to get up about every thirty minutes during the night, one local steambath will bring about normal conditions almost immediately, also in those cases where one is unable to urinate at all.

If necessary this local steambath may be repeated the next day; however, thereafter it should not be used more often than once a week and not for a greater length of time because after the cold sprays, baths, and spongings the body and its organs will be strengthened and put into good working order to take care of its normal functions in the proper manner.

Comments on 4. Scouring Rush Tea

I understand that this tea does not only help improve and heal urinary conditions, it also cleans the stomach, cleans and heals wounds and infections, and stops nose bleeding when sniffed up repeatedly into the nose, for which purposes I have used it with great success.

9

Relieving Hemorrhoids

My husband told me that he had been developing hemorrhoids. At first he did not pay much attention to them, although they were rather annoying. However, when they had broken open, he had to do something about this condition and the following two methods of treatments were applied:

1. BACK COMPRESS:

(see Figure 7 following for correct application)
On Saturday, Monday, and Wednesday, for one week only, for which we provided the following

SUPPLIES:

1. a rubber sheet,
2. a blanket, folded double,
3. two large pillow cases to fit the entire back from the upper neck all the way down to the coccyx (end of spine) and as wide as the shoulders,
4. a bucket with ice-cold water, and followed this

PROCEDURE:

1. covered the bed with the rubber sheet,
2. placed the blanket crosswise on the rubber sheet in such a manner that it would reach from the upper

neck to the legs with the rubber sheet extending an inch or more on top and bottom.

3. placed the two pillow cases on top of each other to form four layers, and dipped them in the water, wringing them out gently—not too dry, but not dripping wet—and put them on the blanket, with the blanket extending an inch or more on top and bottom,

4. fully undressed my husband placed himself squarely on the wet pillow cases, making sure that they reached from the upper neck all the way down to the coccyx,

5. the overhanging sides of the blanket were tucked in well, first the one and then the other, overlapping each other,

6. then he covered himself with the rest of the bedding,

7. after an hour removed the entire compress, including blanket and rubber sheeting,

8. having put on his pajamas as quickly as possible, my husband stayed in bed warmly covered for about another half hour, after which time he dressed completely and went about his regular routine.

2. SITZ BATH:

(Figure 8 shows the correct position)
On Sunday and Tuesday during first week, thereafter once a week for four weeks, for which we made the following

PROVISIONS:

1. the bedroom and bathroom were warm,
2. there was no draft from any window or door,
3. there were two extra blankets on the bed, then prepared the following

SUPPLIES:

1. a round galvanized tub, about the size of four pails, placed inside our bathtub and filled with the coldest water possible,

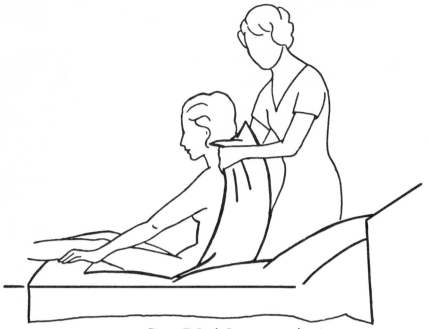

Figure 7: Back Compress application.

2. a bath sheet in readiness,
3. a sweater worn over the pajama top, and followed
   this

PROCEDURE:

1. My husband went to bed to get warm and to have
   the bed warm for his return after the bath,
2. stepped quickly into the bathroom after about
   twenty minutes,
3. rolled up his pajama top and sweater almost to the
   armpits—since the water rises righer in the back,
4. removed the bottom part of his pajamas,
5. stepped into the bathtub and sat down in the round
   tub immediately but slowly with his legs dangling
   out,
6. counted thirty seconds thus: "one and twenty", "two
   and twenty", etc., giving the correct rhythm for
   each second,

7. stepped out at the count of fifty and shook the water off somewhat,
8. without drying, wrapped the bath sheet firmly around his hips, tucking the upper corner inside, and rolled down his pajama top and sweater,
9. went to bed as quickly as possible, covering up well, especially around the hips,
10. after an hour dressed completely and went about his regular routine.

Comments on 1. Back Compress

Although the back compress was very cold at first, soon a comfortable warmth developed. It seemed to reduce the heat and bring better circulation in the inflamed area. We checked the compress after about half an hour to make sure that it did not get too warm; otherwise we should have dipped the pillow cases again into the cold water. This compress also had a beneficial effect on the spine.

Figure 8: Sitz Bath—General positioning.

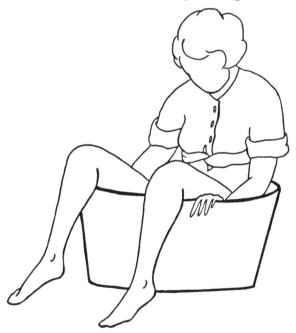

Comments on 2. Sitz Bath

This had a very agreeable and cooling effect which reduced the feeling of pressure. After having gone to bed and covered up warmly, my husband felt a tingling sensation through his entire body, even into his fingertips. He was very much relaxed and felt most comfortable. After a few minutes a well-balanced warmth spread over his whole body. That evening he could even sleep much better.

If he took the sitz bath at night, he usually changed into his pajamas after he had been in bed for half an hour, and went right to sleep.*

GENERAL

With the passing of each day the hemorrhoids improved gradually and a week later they seemed to have gone entirely.

In order to prevent any recurrence, a person may continue taking a sitz bath whenever he felt it necessary, which may be anywhere from once a month to once a year. My husband has never again been bothered with hemorrhoids.

* The sitz bath is not only beneficial in cases of insomnia, but it also eliminates gases, improves the digestion and the bowel activity, and helps the blood circulation in general.

10

Insomnia

My husband from time to time suffered from insomnia, with the result of many restless nights of tossing and turning, getting up again and reading half of the night, trying again, only to fall fitfully asleep toward morning when it was almost time to get up and go to work. He never took any sleeping pills because he tries to stay away from any form of drugs.

Since he had such good results also with regard to insomnia when using the sitz bath for hemorrhoids (see previous chapter), he started taking one of the following water-method applications whenever insomnia starts to manifest itself:

1. SITZ BATH:

One a week, for as many weeks as needed (for details see Chapter 9, 2).

2. FOOT WRAPPINGS or LEG WRAPPINGS:

For one hour at night, not more than three nights a week, whenever needed (for Foot Wrappings see Chapter 13, Case No. 4) (for Leg Wrappings, see Chapter 31, 4).

3. FULL SPONGING:

One or two a night, whenever needed (for details see Chapter 2, Case No. 1).

4. FULL BATH:

(Figures 9 and 10 on next pages show you how to proceed)
One or two a night, not more than three nights a week for
as many weeks as needed, for which he made the following

PROVISIONS:

1. the bathroom and bedroom were warm,
2. there was no draft from any window or door,
3. there were two extra blankets on the bed, arranged
   for the following

SUPPLIES:

1. a tubful of the coldest water possible,
2. a large bath sheet,
3. a bath towel, and followed this

PROCEDURE:

1. stepped into the bathroom as quickly as possible,
2. removed his pajamas,
3. stepped into the tub, sitting down immediately but
   slowly, stretching the legs, then leaning backward
   to get the water up to the neck (if necessary pulled
   up the knees in case of a short tub) completing all
   in about six seconds,
4. stepped out of the tub immediately, shaking off the
   water somewhat,
5. without drying, wrapped the bath sheet from under
   the armpits down to the legs, tucking in one corner
   at the top,
6. draped the bath towel over his shoulders like a cape,
7. ran into bed and covered up well, tucked in loosely
   but well all around from the neck to the feet,
8. on awaking during the night, removed the towels
   and put on his pajamas,
9. if unable to go back to sleep after about half an
   hour, took another bath as before, i.e., repeating 1.
   to 8.

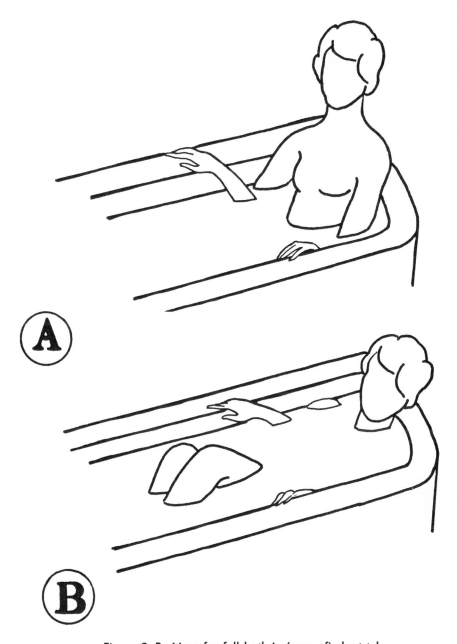

Figure 9: Positions for full bath in (case of) short tub:
A. Sitting up and stretching legs forward.
B. Pulling up knees, leaning back.

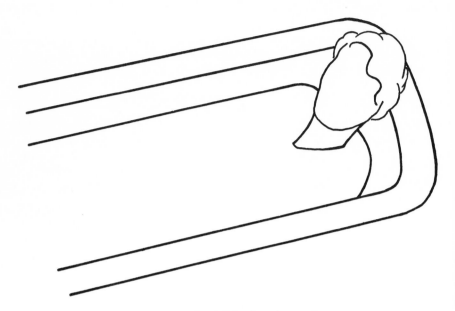

Figure 10: Position for full bath in long tub.

Comments on 1. Sitz Bath

If my husband tossed for more than half an hour, he got up, filled the little tub with cold water and took the sitz bath. This seemed to take the pressure out of his head and relaxed him so completely that he was asleep within ten minutes usually. Often he preferred not to use the bath sheet to wrap around his waist after the bath, but simply put on his pajama pants without having dried himself, since this would more likely assure him of an undisturbed sleep. Thereafter he usually slept soundly the whole night through.

Within a short time his sleeping habits became more normal and the intervals between the baths longer. Sometimes he could go almost an entire year without a sitz bath.

In later years, whenever he felt that the cause for the insomnia was of a different nature, he took one of the other three applications listed previously in this chapter.

Comments on 2. Foot Wrapping

Whenever the foot wrappings seem uncomfortable, you might use wrappings around the leg calf instead with the same good results. This method helps to take the pressure out of your head and to relax you very nicely so that you will soon drop off to sleep. If the feet remain warm, one can sleep with the wrappings on through the night. However, if your feet become cold, remove the wrappings immediately, and drift off to sleep promptly.

Comments on 3. Cold Sponging

After the cold sponging, you will become very much relaxed, so that within a short time you will be fast asleep. However, when my husband awoke too early in the morning, he took another sponging and went right back to sleep. He repeated these the following two evenings and slept well thereafter for quite a while. It seemed that these spongings had brought about a healthy balance of energy in his working body system, and they can do the same for you.

Comments on 4. Full Bath

As a rule my husband prefers a cold full bath to the cold sponging because he gets through with it faster. However, before getting out of bed he realizes that as little time as possible should be lost between getting out of bed and stepping into the tub. Therefore, once he has made up his mind to go through with it, he does not hesitate in front of the tub, knowing that it is important for the body to remain warm.

Nothing seems to relax him so completely as a cold full bath. It is amazing how quickly he goes to sleep after having taken one. It seems to balance his whole system and also keep him more relaxed during his working hours. One cold bath would usually let him sleep all night through. Only rarely would he have to take another one later in the night. After having taken the bath for two or three more nights, he could usually sleep regularly and soundly for a long period.

GENERAL

Of course, the reasons for insomnia vary greatly, and many an illness robs a person of his sleep. I have found that by applying the appropriate cold-water applications for a certain illness, thereby assisting the body to cure itself, these applications took care of my insomnia at the same time, letting me sleep soundly during the entire night.

11

Getting Rid of
Unpleasant Mucus

For many years I had been annoyed with the unpleasantness of mucus in my throat, especially in the morning. To improve this condition I took the following applications:

1. UPPER SPRAY:

(Figures 11 and 12 on the next pages show you the direction and position of the water spray.)
Three times a week, for two weeks, for which I made the following

PROVISIONS:

1. the bedroom and bathroom were warm,
2. there was no draft from any door or window,
3. there were two extra blankets on my bed, and arranged the following

SUPPLIES:

1. a rubber hose (or handspray without the spray head) attached to the bathtub faucet,
2. a bathing cap,
3. a bath towel to tuck around my waist,

4. a bath towel to be draped over my shoulders after the spray,
5. the wash basin filled with the coldest possible water and a facecloth in it.

Since I felt chilly, I went to bed first to get comfortably warm. After about twenty minutes I followed this

PROCEDURE:

1. I stepped quickly into the bathroom,
2. put on the bathing cap and removed my pajama top,
3. tucked the bath towel around my waist and bent over the tub with my hands resting on the bottom of it,
4. asked my husband to spray my back thus:
   a. start at the right hand, holding the hose about three inches away, go up the right arm to the shoulder, holding the spray at such an angle that the water covers my whole arm like a sheet, continue further up (since I was bending down) to my waist, covering mainly the right side of my back with the water and letting it flow over the entire back like a sheet for up to thirty seconds, then go back down the way you came up,
   b. start at the left hand, go up the left arm to the shoulder, continue to the waist, hold about thirty seconds, the same as on the right side, and then back again,
5. sponged my chest quickly with the facecloth and cold water,
6. dried my face and hands only,
7. without drying my chest and back, I put the dry bath towel around my shoulders like a cape,
8. removed the bathing cap and the towel from my waist and went quickly to bed, covering up well, the blankets tucked in especially around my shoulders and alongside my arms,
9. got up after an hour and dressed, keeping moderately active for a while.

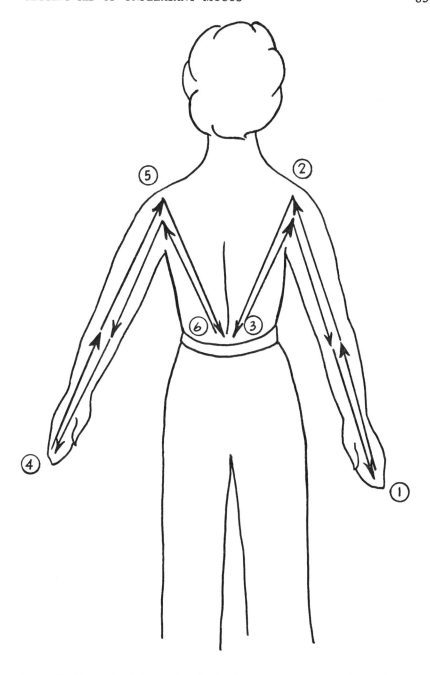

Figure 11: Upper Back Spray for eliminating mucus. Arrows indicate direction of spray application.

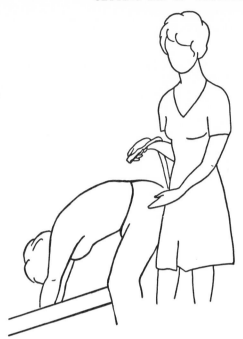

Figure 12: Position for Upper Back Spray. (See also Figure 11)

2. KNEE SPRAY:

(Figure 13 on page 86 gives the directions of the spray. Figure 14 shows the position to be taken during the spray.) Four or five times a week, for four weeks, and at least three times a week thereafter, for which I arranged as

SUPPLY:

a rubber hose (or handspray without the spray head) attached to the bathtub faucet and followed this

PROCEDURE:

1. I removed my shoes and stockings,
2. stepped otherwise fully dressed into the empty bathtub,
3. sprayed my legs with the coldest water possible by holding the hose about three inches away in such a fashion that the water covered the entire leg like a sheet, never in trickles,

    a. starting at the heel of my right leg, at No. 1, and going slowly up to the kneebend, to No. 2, then slowly down again to the heel, to No. 1,

    b. starting at the heel of the left leg at No. 3, and going slowly up to the kneebend, to No. 4, then down again, to No. 3,

    c. repeating a. and b. four times, right, left, right, left, etc.

    d. turning around and starting at the toes of my right leg, No. 1, again going slowly up to the knee, No. 2, and then down again to the toes, No. 1,

    e. starting at the toes of my left leg, No. 3, going slowly up to the knee, No. 4, and down again, No. 3,

    f. repeating d. and e. also four times, right, left, right, left, etc., and completing the whole procedure in about two minutes,

4. without drying my legs, either went to bed and covered up warmly for about half an hour, or put on my stockings and shoes and walked around until my legs were dry and warm.

Comments on 1. Upper Spray

Before getting out of bed for the spray I made it clear to myself that as little time as possible should be lost once I had left the bed, until I started the spray. Therefore once I had made up my mind to go through with it, I did not hesitate in front of the tub, knowing that it is imporant for the body to remain warm.

Since I had no serious lung ailment or heart trouble, I could start right away with the full upper spray; otherwise I should have applied instead an upper sponging for the first few days (for details see Chapter 8, Case No. 1, III) and then started with a very light upper spray.

At first I could take the spray only for a few seconds, but soon was able to take the full thirty seconds on each side.

As soon as I was covered up in bed I developed a very pleasant warmth all through the upper part of my body and could feel it

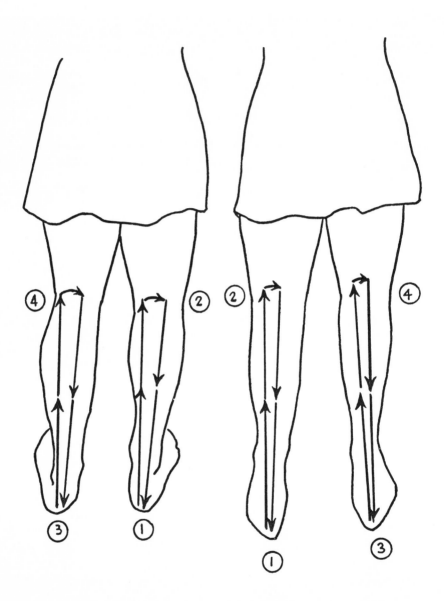

Figure 13: Knee Spray—Arrows indicate direction of spray flow.

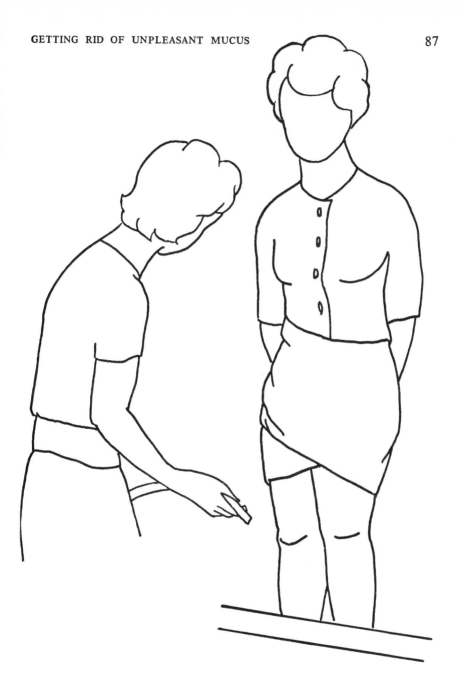

Figure 14: Position for Knee Spray by another. (See also Figure 13)

even in my fingertips. My chest felt as if it were expanding, my breathing was very deep and strong, and the mucus seemed to be getting loose. For the next few days it appeared as if the amount of mucus had increased. I even had to cough during the night. But this was only a general housecleaning, and after awhile I was absolutely free of all mucus and have never been bothered with it since. It also seemed as if my voice had improved.

Comments on 2. Knee Spray

At first I could stand the cold water only three times up and down my legs, but increased it soon. I also found that it was easier to take if I first went very quickly up and down the legs before starting with the regular spray.

The knee spray seemed to balance my blood circulation and draw the blood into the feet, as an important supplement to the concentrated action of the upper spray.

I had always suffered greatly from cold feet, but soon my feet started getting gradually warmer, and today I rarely have cold feet.

You will find that the knee spray furthermore hardens and strengthens the whole body, increases resistance, body warmth, improves bladder, kidneys and other organs, draws the blood away from the head and also the heart, thereby easing the heart activity, and is even beneficial for the throat. I have taken it regularly for the last thirty years.

A Warning for Heart-Trouble Cases

Persons with heart trouble should first walk barefoot for a few days, then walk in cold water for a few additional days (for details see Chapter 13, Case No. 1) and finally start with a short knee spray. Heart patients should check with their doctor if they have any doubts whatever as to the effect of water applications.

12

Relieving Constipation

For about ten years I had suffered from constipation until I started applying cold water in the following manner:

1. HIP SPRAY:

Twice during first week, once a week thereafter (for details see Chapter 7, Case No. 1).

2. HALF BATH:

One during first week, two during second week (see TONSILLITIS, Chapter 6).

3. BACK SPRAY:

(Figures 15 and 16 on the following pages give you the directions and positions)
Three times during first week, once during second week, for which I made the following

PROVISIONS:

1. the bedroom and bathroom were warm,
2. there was no draft from any door or window,
3. there were two extra blankets on the bed, and arranged for the following

SUPPLIES:

1. a rubber hose (or handspray without the spray head) attached to the bathtub faucet,
2. a bath sheet,
3. a bath towel,
and followed this

PROCEDURE:

1. Since I felt chilly I went to bed for about twenty minutes to get comfortably warm,
2. went quickly into the bathroom and undressed completely without losing too much time,
3. stepped into the empty bathtub and asked my husband to spray my back as follows, holding the hose about three inches away in such a fashion that the water covers like a sheet, never in trickles:
   a. start at the right heel (see Figure 15 at No. 1) and proceed up the leg to the hip (to No. 2) then down again,
   b. start at the left heel (at No. 3) proceeding again up the leg to the hip (to No. 4), but do *not* go down again; instead,
   c. go over to the right hip (to No. 2) and proceed up the back to the right shoulder (to No. 5) (but not so high that the water runs down the front), then down again to the right hip (to No. 2) and then over to the left hip (to No. 4),
   d. proceed from the left hip (No. 4) up the back to the left shoulder (to No. 6), then all the way down to the left heel (to No. 3)
   e. repeat the entire procedure twice, i.e., from a. to d.,
4. without drying myself I wrapped the bath sheet around me from under the armpits to the legs, tucking in one corner at the top,
5. draped the bath towel over my shoulders like a cape,
6. ran into bed and covered up well, tucked in all over,

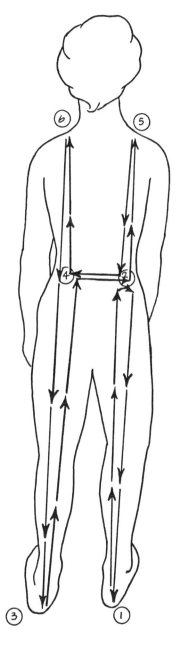

Figure 15: Back Spray for constipation. Arrows and area numbers indicate spray flow pattern.

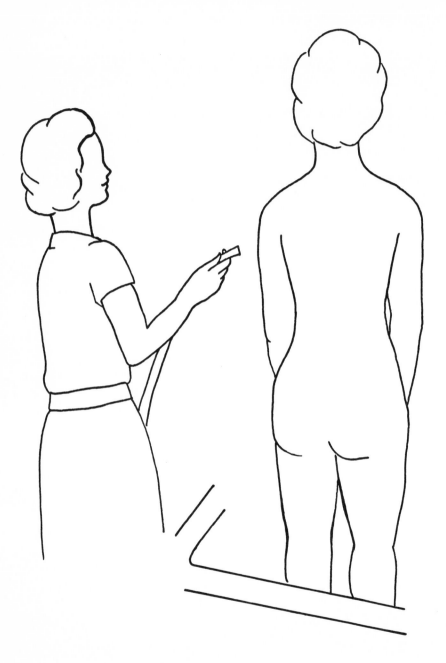

Figure 16: Position for Back Spray. (See also Figure 15)

7. after half an hour removed the towels and put on my pajamas, staying in bed for another half hour, after which time I dressed and went about my regular routine.

4. FULL SPRAY:

(Figure 17 following gives the directions of the spray. Figure 18 shows the position to be taken during the spray.)
One spray during second week, one during third week, for which I made the following

PROVISIONS:

The same as under 3. Back Spray, arranged for the following

SUPPLIES:

The same as under 3. Back Spray, and followed this

PROCEDURE:

1. the same as under 3. BACK SPRAY,
2. ditto,
3. from a. to d.: ditto (but *not* repeating e),
4. turned around and sprayed myself thus:
   a. starting at the right toes (see Fig. 18 at No. 1) and proceeding up the leg to the right side of my stomach (to No. 2), then down again,
   b. starting at the left toes (at No. 3) proceeding up the leg to the left side of my stomach (to No. 4), but *not* down again, instead
   c. swinging over to the right side of the stomach (to No. 2) and continuing up to the right shoulder (to No. 5), then down again to the right side of the stomach (to No. 2) and then over to the left side of the stomach (to No. 4),
   d. proceeding from the left side of the stomach (No. 4) up to the left shoulder (to No. 6), then all the way down to the left toes (to No. 3).
5. having finished spraying in less than three minutes,

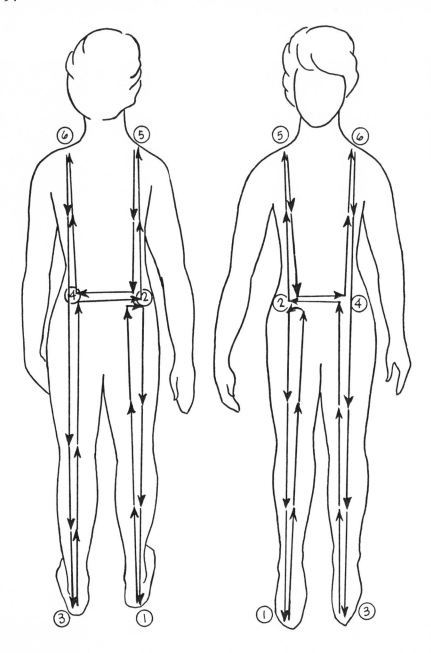

Figure 17: Full Spray—Arrows and body area numbers indicate spray flow
pattern.

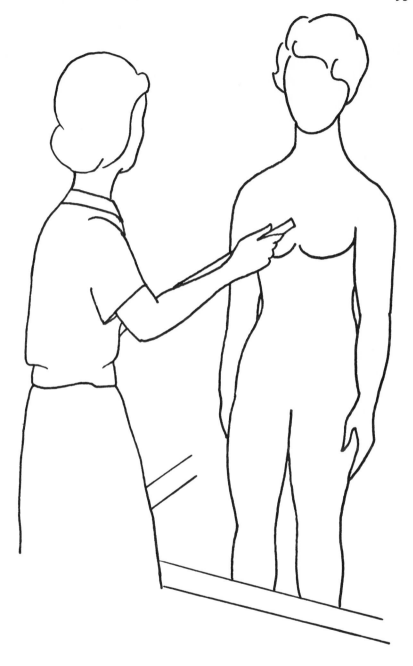

Figure 18: Position for Full Spray. (See also Figure 17)

without drying myself, I wrapped the bath sheet around me from under the armpits down to the legs, tucking in one corner at the top,

6. draped the bath towel over my shoulders like a cape,
7. ran into bed and covered up well, tucked in all around,
8. after half an hour removed the towels and put on my pajamas, stayed in bed for another half hour, after which time I dressed and went about my regular routine.

Comments on 1. Hip Spray

Even while spraying I felt the blood circulating through my legs, apparently in an effort to fight off the cold water, making my skin look pink. After I was wrapped up warmly in bed I felt a tingling sensation all through my legs and body, even into my fingertips, although the rest of my body had not been sprayed. My breathing was deep and pleasant, and I felt completely relaxed.

The hip spray is not only beneficial to the bowels but to a great extent also to the kidneys, liver, bladder and all other parts of the abdomen, having a healing influence also on hemorrhoids.

Comments on 2. Half Bath

After I was wrapped up well in bed I felt a great warmth surging through my whole body; my breathing again was deep and I felt completely relaxed (see also Comments under TONSILLITIS, Chapter 6).

Comments on 3. Back Spray

The first time I was able to take the back spray only once. After I was back in bed I was sorry I did not have it three times, because I felt immediately warm and comfortable; also during the next spray I found that the second and third round of the spray is much easier to take than the first.

This spray seems to regulate the blood circulation and is very invigorating, strengthening, increasing the body warmth and accordingly very beneficial to all organs of the body. Except for the first week, it should not be taken more than once a week.

Comments on 4. Full Spray

I took this spray after I had accustomed myself to cold water by the various partial sprays, since it is advisable to get the body gradually used to cold water. For this full spray it is especially important that the entire body feel warm before taking it.

For this spray, the same as for all other cold-water applications, I made it clear to myself, before getting out of bed for the spray, that as little time as possible should be lost once I had left the bed until I started the spray. Therefore, when I had made up my mind to go through with it, I did not hesitate in front of the tub, knowing that it is important for the body to remain warm.

After I was back in bed I felt a tingling over my entire body and very soon an agreeable warmth and a feeling of great well-being. The spray tended to increase my blood circulation beneficially, strengthen the vitality of the whole system, improve the rate of body warmth, tone up the system and increase its natural resistance to disease.

The reaction is entirely different from taking an ordinary cold shower. Since the full spray is started at the feet, the blood seems to be drawn to the feet first, away from the heart and head, thereby increasing the circulation and body warmth, and I did not have the unpleasant feeling of having to catch my breath when the cold water reached my chest, as I would have to do if the cold water hit me first from over my head. Instead the cold water came gradually up the back, first one side and then the other, and the same in front. I had a definite feeling that my blood circulation was thereby being evenly distributed over my whole body, stimulating all organs to their proper functioning.

GENERAL

I had discontinued all laxatives when starting the cold-water applications, and after three days I had my first normal bowel movement, then every two days for about a week, and daily thereafter, without ever using a laxative again for more than 30 years. However, I must add that ever since that time I have taken one or the other cold-water applications at least once a week, and also knee and arm sprays four or five times a week. Furthermore, I have improved my diet by reducing the intake of sweets and starches, and adding more green vegetables, fruit, and whole wheat bread.

These water applications may also alleviate and even prevent gout (arthritis) and assist the "total body" in curing this disease eventually.

13

Taking Care of Feet
and Ankles

The secret of having strong and healthy feet lies in having them properly toughened and hardened. They should never be pampered by heating pads, hot water bottles, heavy furlined shoes, or thick slippers. It only weakens them and at the same time casts a negative influence on the efficiency of the whole system of the body's functioning.

If you start walking barefoot as described under Case No. 1, following, even if it is only for a few minutes each day, after a few days you will experience how much better not only your feet but you yourself feel. If you do not have a garden or backyard where you can walk barefoot in the summer, even walking barefoot on the bare floor in your own room for a few minutes every night before you go to bed will be very helpful. But you have to keep walking constantly; never stand still in one spot. The feet have to have action. Once you feel the beneficial effect on your feet, you will want to do more and walk in cold water as outlined in Case No. 1 as follows:

CASE No. 1: FEET SUFFERING UNDULY FROM COLD AND STRAIN

The winter of 1934 was the last season I suffered greatly from cold feet, as I had done every previous winter. My circulation was so poor that it seemed as if I had no blood at all in my feet. As a child I used to wear long woolen stockings and often took a hot-water bottle to bed at night to get my feet warm. But the more I used the hot-water bottle, the more my feet lost their own warmth. Since I had learned that cold water would cure this condition, I developed the following two methods:

1. WALK IN COLD WATER:

(Figure 19 following demonstrates the method.)
Every evening before going to bed for two weeks, for which I arranged the following

SUPPLY:

I filled the tub with the coldest water possible
a. the first day high enough to cover my ankles,
b. each subsequent day a little higher, until finally the capacity of the tub was reached, and followed this

PROCEDURE:

1. I changed into a warm night gown plus bathrobe,
2. walked up and down in the bathtub
   a. the first day for one minute,
   b. each subsequent day a little longer until I was able to hold out for five minutes,
3. always stepped out as soon as my feet started to feel warm, because I knew I should not wait until they started to feel cold again,
4. without drying my feet, went to bed immediately and stayed there for the night.

2. WALKING BAREFOOT:

Daily whenever possible, all life long, for which I made the following

PROVISIONS:

1. that I was properly dressed and felt warm otherwise,

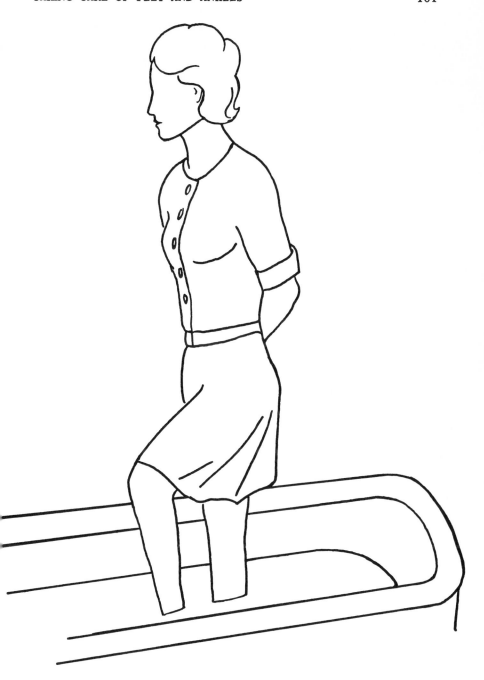

Figure 19: Position for walking in cold water in the bathtub.

2. that I kept walking briskly in cold weather and did not sit or stand still in my bare feet on a cold floor even in warm weather, and according to conditions and circumstances alternated the

PROCEDURE:

1. by either walking in the house as long as comfortable,
2. or by walking in wet grass up to half an hour, depending on the temperature, followed, without drying the feet, by a walk in shoes and stockings until feet were warm and dry,
3. or by walking on wet stones, proceeding the same as under 2.,
4. or by walking in newly fallen snow (*never* in old snow), for five minutes, followed, without drying of feet, by a walk in shoes and stockings until my feet were warm and dry.

Comments on 1. Walk in Cold Water

When I first stepped into the cold water, it was rather painful and I felt the penetrating cold, but soon my feet started to feel numb and then warm. At that moment I knew that the cold water had done its job and induced warmth, and I stepped out immediately before my feet had a chance to get cold again, went quickly to bed, where my feet became almost burning warm. I felt very light, and even my breathing seemed to be easier; my heart beat more quietly. After having walked in cold water for almost two weeks, my whole system seemed to be strengthened with beneficial effects on the bladder and kidney, stomach gases and even headaches.

Comments on 2. Walking Barefoot

Since my feet did not suffer from broken skin or perspiration, it was safe for me to walk in the snow.

I have been walking barefoot daily for over thirty years and find my feet in excellent condition. I never suffer from cold feet. I can wear all sorts of shoes, whether high or low heels, and never suffer from strain, or burning or swollen feet, even if I walk for hours.

Whenever I walk barefoot, my head feels light. It also seems to have a calming effect, even on the stomach, and especially on the heart. I believe that it has not only toughened my feet, but my whole system, and has helped to establish a good balance in my nervous system. My blood circulation seems to be much improved, I am less susceptible to colds, and my bladder seems to be strengthened.

I like to mention here that my two daughters always removed their shoes and socks as soon as they entered the house, from early childhood on, and in the country they walked barefoot all day long whenever the weather permitted. It is not surprising therefore that they both have strong feet, a good blood circulation, and are little susceptible to colds. When my oldest daughter had her physical examination upon entering college, the attending physician not only gave her the highest rating for excellent health, but also exclaimed that she had the healthiest looking pair of feet he had ever seen. My two daughters are married now, and their own children also walk barefoot at every opportunity, and enjoy very good health.

CASE No. 2: SWOLLEN FEET

A friend of mine had been suffering from swollen feet for a number of years. One day she asked me what she could do about it. I outlined the applications to her which I should take in such a case, as follows:

1. FULL SPONGING WITH VINEGAR-WATER:

Twice a week, for three weeks—see Chapter 2—with the following exception under

SUPPLIES:

2. a basin filled with half water and half vinegar.

2. VINEGAR-COMPRESS ON ABDOMEN:

Twice a week, for three weeks (see Chapter 17, Case No. 1)

3. KNEE SPRAY:

Every other day, for three weeks, at least twice a week thereafter (see Chapter 11, 2).

4. HIP SPRAY:

Every other day, alternating with knee spray, for three weeks, once a week thereafter (see Chapter 7, Case No. 1).

5. THREE HERB TEA MIXTURES:

One cupful daily, taken in three portions, morning, noon, and night, for three weeks (see Chapter 39, 5).

6. HAY-FLOWER FOOT WRAPPING:

One every other day, for one week, one a week during second and third week.

SUPPLIES:

1. to one and a half tablespoonfuls of hay-flower in a bowl add one and a half quarts of boiling water, cover and let steep for five to ten minutes,
2. one kitchen towel for each foot,
3. one face towel for each foot,
4. one small piece of plastic for each foot.

PROCEDURE:

(for each foot separately)

1. Dip the kitchen towel into the warm, strained or unstrained hay-flower tea, wring out carefully (not too dry, but not dripping wet) and wrap around the foot and ankle very carefully so that the towel clings closely to the foot all around, but not too tight in order not to interfere with the blood circulation,
2. wrap the face towel over the wet towel in such a manner that the wet towel is completely hidden, then cover with the plastic and the bedding,
3. after an hour remove the wrappings and dip the wet

towels again, this time in the cold solution, repeating
1. and 2.,
4. after the second hour remove the entire wrappings
   and keep the feet warm in bed for another hour.

Comments on 6. Foot Wrapping

This wrapping lets you sleep restfully and refreshingly. If you
fall asleep before the hour is up, you do not need to remove the
wrapping until you wake up, when it has to be taken off immediately. It takes all tiredness out of the feet, reduces the pain and
swelling, unless the cause for the swelling lies in the condition of
the entire system, in which case it is necessary to apply cold water
to the whole body and thereby improve its condition. The foot and
leg wrappings are also very beneficial for the ears and tend to
improve the quality of hearing.

CASE No. 3: SPRAINED ANKLE

My husband sprained his ankle very badly while skiing. It was
so painful that he suspected a fracture. However, according to the
X-rays this was not the case.

In order to ease the pain and reduce the swelling we applied
the following:

1. ANKLE WRAPPING:

One a day, for four days, for which he arranged the following

SUPPLIES:

1. a bowl of cold water with about six ice cubes
2. a kitchen towel, folded twice into four layers, to fit
   around the ankle,
3. a face towel, folded once lengthwise, to wrap around
   the compress, and followed this

PROCEDURE:

1. placed the folded face towel underneath the ankle,
2. dipped the folded kitchen towel into the cold water
   and wrung it out gently, not too dry but not dripping
   wet,

3. placed the wet kitchen towel on top of the face towel underneath the ankle.

4. folded one side of the kitchen towel over the ankle, lightly but close enough to cling to it, then the other side,

5. wrapped the face towel around the compress, extending about an inch beyond the kitchen towel on both ends in order to keep any draft out,

6. after ten minutes dipped kitchen towel again into the cold water and proceeded as before,

7. every fifteen minutes thereafter dipped kitchen towel into the cold water and proceeded as before,

8. after altogether one and a half hours removed the entire compress and kept foot covered and warm for about an hour,

9. applied light bandage on ankle for support in walking.

2. KNEE SPRAY:

One every morning, for two weeks (for details see Chapter 11, 2, also Comments). While spraying he always held the hose an extra three or four seconds on the sprained ankle, both on the way up and the way down.

Comments on 1. Ankle Wrapping

The cold compress had a very soothing effect, reduced the pain gradually, and at the end of the first hour and a half the swelling had gone down considerably so that my husband could walk carefully with a cane. Every day there was a marked improvement, and after four days of water applications he could walk without a cane.

Comments on 2. Knee Spray

The knee sprays were also beneficial in reducing the pain and swelling. They tended to improve the blood circulation generally, and particularly in the legs and ankle, thereby strengthening the sprained ankle considerably so that it has never been a source of complaint again.

CASE No. 4: WEAK ANKLES

During the first thirty years of my life I always suffered from very weak ankles. My feet turned over quite frequently, and often I sprained one or the other of my ankles. Therefore I always had to walk carefully when wearing high heels.

The following water applications gave my ankles adequate strength for any demands I made upon them.

1. KNEE SPRAY:

Four or five days each week, for as many weeks as necessary (for details see Chapter 11, 2, also Comments).

2. FOOT WRAPPING:

Once a week, for as many weeks as necessary, for which I arranged the following

SUPPLIES:

1. two kitchen towels
2. two face towels or heavy socks
3. a bowl of ice-cold water and followed this

PROCEDURE:

1. I dipped each kitchen towel into the cold water, wrung it out lightly, not too dry, but not dripping wet, and wrapped one such towel around each foot and ankle very carefully so that the towel would cling to the foot closely all around, but not tight enough to interfere with the blood circulation,
2. wrapped a face towel or wore a large woolen sock over the wet towel of each foot, covered with bedding,
3. after an hour removed the entire wrappings and kept my feet warm in bed for at least an hour. Whenever I applied the wrappings before retiring for the night, I went to sleep soon afterward and removed all wrappings when I woke up, whether during the night or in the morning.

Comments on 1. Knee Spray

As I applied the knee sprays regularly my feet and ankles improved gradually and soon became so strong that I started to go skiing, without ever having any trouble with my ankles. I am able to go on long hikes even in rough territory and have never twisted or sprained my ankles since. I can now walk very easily in high heels and still go ice skating, although I am over sixty.

In addition, the knee sprays have improved my blood circulation so that my feet are always warm. The wonderful experience I have had with the cold sprays is that they were always good for my whole body, they apparently improved the condition of my bladder and kidneys, my headaches have disappeared almost entirely, and I have never had tonsillitis again. The knee sprays have toughened my entire system and strengthened it.

Comments on 2. Foot Wrapping

Whenever I applied the foot wrappings before retiring for the night, I slept very soundly. Also, the wrappings took all tiredness out of my feet, which became very warm afterward and remained warm longer in general.

The wrappings took all pain out of my feet and reduced any swelling. They even helped greatly in the case of tonsillitis.

Foot wrappings are beneficial for alleviating gout (arthritis), also for the health of the ears, and to improve the hearing, especially if wrappings are dipped into a warm hay-flower solution (for details see Chapter 8, Case No. 1, 4, HAYFLOWER COMPRESS). Furthermore, the wrappings are helpful for pneumonia and other inflamations if dipped into a cold solution of half water and half vinegar, but have to be dipped again and repeated as soon as feet get hot. However, should feet get cold after a while, the wrappings have to be removed.

14

Getting Rid of Lumbago

It is amazing how a very painful ailment like lumbago can sometimes be cured with a very simple remedy like water and vinegar within a few hours. The following three cases will tell you how this application works for overcoming lumbago.

CASE No. 1

One afternoon my husband had gone ice skating. He was skating around the pond at a good pace, bending forward for greater speed, when someone crossed his path and he had to make an unexpected stop, which caused him to straighten out suddenly. At that moment he felt as if something had snapped in his back, which was extremely painful unless he remained in the bent-over position. There was nothing else for him to do but to walk to our house nearby in this bent-over position. I helped him undress and get into bed.

He had crawled into bed on all fours and rolled in sideways with the greatest care and difficulty, assisted by my support. When lying flat on his back he was somewhat relieved, and I covered him up warmly.

I offered to give him one of the following applications (either would be quite sufficient):

1. BACK SPONGING (WITH WARM WATER AND VINEGAR):

One every hour, repeated as often as needed, for which I arranged the following

SUPPLIES:

1. a bowl with two cups of vinegar and two cups of hot water,
2. a good-size facecloth, and followed this

PROCEDURE:

1. Standing at the right side of the bed, I rolled my husband on his left side with the greatest of care (since he was unable to turn by himself),
2. dipped the facecloth in the warm vinegar solution, squeezing it out just lightly, and washed my husband's entire back in even strokes, as fast and thoroughly as I could
   a. starting at his left shoulder and going all the way down his back, including the thigh,
   b. after having dipped the cloth again starting at the neck and going all the way down the middle to the coccyx (end of the spine),
   c. after having dipped the cloth again starting at his right shoulder and going all the way down again (including the thigh),
3. without drying him, rolled him flat on his back and covered him up, tucked in well—especially around the shoulders and along the sides.
4. after one hour, repeated 1. to 3. with the vinegar solution warmed up,
5. after another hour my husband got dressed warmly and went about his usual routine in a moderate way.

2. BACK COMPRESS (WITH WARM WATER AND VINEGAR):

(See Figure 7 in Chapter 9 for correct application)
One every hour for three hours, repeated the next day if necessary, for which I provided the following

SUPPLIES:

1. a rubber sheet,
2. a blanket,
3. two large pillow cases to fit the entire back, from the upper neck all the way down to the end of the spine and as wide as the shoulders,
4. a bowl with two cups of hot water and two cups of vinegar, and followed this

PROCEDURE:

1. line the bed with the rubber sheet,
2. place the blanket, folded double, crosswise on the rubber sheet to reach from the upper neck to the legs, with the rubber sheet extending about an inch on top and bottom,
3. place the two pillow cases on top of each other to form four layers and dip in the warm vinegar solution, wring out gently (not too dry, but not dripping wet) and place on the blanket, with the blanket extending about an inch on top and bottom,
4. fully undressed, my husband to lay with his back squarely on the wet pillow cases, the latter to reach from the upper neck down to the coccyx.
5. fold over the overhanging sides of the blanket, first one and then the other, overlapping each other,
6. cover well with the regular bedding,
7. after one hour repeat 3. to 6. if necessary, dipping the pillow cases in the cold vinegar solution,
8. after another hour repeat 3. to 6. again if necessary, dipping the pillow cases in the cold vinegar solution,
9. after the last compress is on for one hour, remove it in its entirety, put on pajamas and cover up warmly for another hour.

Comments on 1. Back Sponging

After the first sponging my husband felt relaxed, with a prickling sensation all over his back. When the first hour was over, he was already able to turn by himself on his left side, although slowly and very carefully, since there was still some pain connected with it. A single sponging had already enabled him to move that much.

After the second sponging and the second hour, all pain was gone. It may seem incredible, but my husband got up carefully and dressed himself, without any discomfort. You may hardly believe that this was the end of the lumbago, but it actually never came back. I am certain that we had such a quick result because we did not lose any time after the onset in applying the sponging. I had expected to make at least three or four spongings, but prompt action with water applications usually gives benefits very quickly.

Comments on 2. Back Compress

If the back spongings had not brought the desired result in such a short time, we should have applied the back compress, which I firmly believe would also have done away with the lumbago. If we had started with the back compress and if afterward a slight discomfort was left, then a sponging as outlined before would easily have taken care of it.

CASE No. 2

One summer my husband took a quick trip north to check on our ski cabin in the White Mountains. A friend of ours had started building his house on the opposite corner. When my husband arrived, this friend was in bed flat on his back with great lumbago pains. He told my husband that while he was pouring the cement blocks (he was making his own) he had apparently strained himself and had to stop working immediately because of the great pain in his back. My husband then suggested to him (while telling him of his own experience) a *BACK SPONGING* (with warm water and vinegar) (for details see Case No. 1, 1) and explained to him how to have it done.

The next morning when my husband went to find out how his friend was, he was happy to see him busy pouring his cement blocks. He kept on working without any further pains.

CASE No. 3

One day the boss of my old company came into my office and was apparently in great pain. When he told me that he had lumbago and was going home because of the pain, I mentioned to him the *BACK COMPRESS* (with warm water and vinegar) (for details see Case No. 1, 2) and gave him a short description of how to apply it, although I was very doubtful whether he would try it. He seemed to listen only with one ear and left almost immediately. I felt that I had at least done my duty and shared my experience with him, so that he could benefit from it if he so desired.

The next morning I was greatly and very pleasantly surprised to see him in the office again with a happy smile and saying to me: "I did it, and it helped."

15

Taking the Worry Out of Pregnancy

I became pregnant at the age of thirty. Since my only sister had had a most difficult time at twenty and a delivery so very dangerous that she could never have another child, I wanted to make certain that with me everything would take its normal course. Therefore I programmed myself to take regularly a

HALF BATH:

One every other day, for nine months (see TONSILLITIS, Chapter 6, 3) with

PROVISIONS:

(the same as Chapter 6, 3)

SUPPLIES:

(the same as Chapter 6, 3)

PROCEDURE:

1. to 4. (the same as Chapter 6, 3),
5. just stretched my legs for one second,
6. stepped out of the tub after about two seconds, shaking the water off somewhat,
7. to 9. (the same as Chapter 6, 3).

Comments

Since I was not certain whether the usual ten-second half bath would be in order, I limited myself to only two seconds. I continued these half baths up to the day the baby was born.

All through the nine months I felt well and kept up my usual activities without any restrictions, except that I discontinued playing tennis. There was never the slightest danger of a miscarriage. These half baths will work to strengthen the organs and generally tend to prevent a possibility of miscarriage.

During my regular visits to the doctor's office I was happy to learn that all tests were very satisfactory, even the urine tests were in order, despite the fact that I had had bladder and also kidney trouble for a number of years. This only confirmed my conviction that the cold-water applications (see Chapter 8, Case No. 1) had cured me. My health was excellent. I did not even have swollen ankles and was never restricted in my diet. The delivery was normal, and I had a very healthy and always very hungry baby.

When I was expecting my second baby, I followed the same procedure with the same excellent results.

16

Getting Rid of Laryngitis

During one winter, a friend of ours stayed overnight with us. When he arrived he could hardly talk above a whisper and was very much concerned about a very important business appointment he had the following day, as sales representative. It was apparent that under the prevailing condition the success of this meeting was somewhat in doubt. He needed help quickly and was in a state of mind in which he would have tried anything.

I mentioned to him that if I were in his place, I should take one of the following applications, and if the condition remained chronic, then all four types of applications below should be utilized to cover all phases of the laryngitis attack.

1. HIP SPRAY:

One in late afternoon, if necessary repeated on three successive days (for details see Chapter 7, Case No. 1).

2. BACK SPRAY:

One in evening, if necessary repeated on three successive days (for details see Chapter 12, 3).

3. HALF BATH:

One in the morning, if necessary repeated on two successive days (see TONSILLITIS, Chapter 6, 3).

4. THROAT WRAPPING:

One at night, if necessary repeated the following night (see TONSILLITIS, Chapter 6, 1).

Comments on 3. Half Bath

Our suffering friend decided to try the Half-Bath application, which he took at night as directed, before retiring. He slept well through the night and the next morning to his great surprise and joy his voice was functioning normally again. It was incredible to him that a single half bath should have brought his voice back. He told us that he had been rather skeptical, but he figured that he had nothing to lose. I am happy to say that he went to his meeting as scheduled and his voice remained intact in carrying out his meeting duties.

The half bath had taken the blocking blood pressure away from his throat, brought a better circulation and also relaxed him to enable his normal body functions to do their curative work. The half bath had had such a quick result because he had taken it right at the onset of his laryngitis.

17

Stopping Diarrhea and Vomiting

Diarrhea itself can sometimes be a necessary internal body cleansing method, in which case it would not be advisable to stop it suddenly by any medicine. However, the methods outlined under Cases No. 1 and No. 2 in this chapter can have only beneficial results because they strengthen the body and assist it in getting rid of any poisons or impurities, at the same time helping it to return to normal health and vigor in a very short time.

CASE No. 1: ACUTE DIARRHEA AND VOMITING

When my little daughter was just two years old she had a severe case of vomiting and diarrhea. She had never been ill before, and I did not know whether I could apply the cold-water methods at her young age. We had a very excellent pediatrician to whom I used to take her for regular check-ups. When the vomiting continued into the second day I telephoned him, and he came and examined her, prescribing some medicine which I gave her regularly as directed. Unfortunately the medicine did not stay in her stomach long enough to do any good. The doctor had also given me a very strict diet for her, but not even plain water stayed in her stomach, with the result that after two days her body became dehydrated so that her skin started to wrinkle. Her hands looked like those of an old person, she was a very pitiful sight. I was ex-

tremely worried, and decided to place my faith in water application
as follows:

VINEGAR-WATER COMPRESS ON THE ABDOMEN:

One a day for two days, if necessary repeated every other day
for two weeks, for which I arranged the following

PROVISIONS:

1. a small kitchen towel folded twice into four layers,
   to cover her entire abdomen, including the stomach,
2. a bath towel,
3. a bowl with one cup of hot water and one cup of
   vinegar (in case of a rash, less vinegar is used) and
   followed this

PROCEDURE:

1. I put my little girl to bed with a sweater over her
   nightgown for added warmth, and rolled up her
   night gown to her chest,
2. dipped the folded kitchen towel into the warm
   vinegar solution, wrung it out carefully, neither too
   dry nor dripping wet, and placed it gently but firmly
   on her abdomen so that it would cling to her body,
3. covered the compress with the folded bath towel in
   such a way that the bath towel would extend about
   an inch on all sides,
4. covered her up well with the regular bedding, especially tucked in around her hips,
5. after thirty minutes dipped the folded kitchen towel
   again, this time into the cool solution, and proceeded the same as under 2., 3., and 4.,
6. after another thirty minutes removed the entire
   compress and kept her well covered with the bedding
   for another hour, after which time I dressed her
   and allowed her to get up.

Comments

When I told my little girl about preparing a compress for her
stomach, she was really too weak to object, and when I finally

placed it on her abdomen, she seemed to like it. The wet warmth must have felt good, and she was very much relaxed. In a few minutes I could see that her eyes were getting sleepy, and soon she was sound asleep. I had come prepared to show her pictures and toys, or to sing to her, in order to keep her very quiet and well covered, but since she fell asleep I just sat with her so that she would not uncover herself in her sleep.

When I renewed the compress she awoke for a moment, but went right back to sleep. She did not even awake when I finally removed the entire compress very carefully, but slept for almost two hours. I had stayed at her bedside the entire time to be sure that she remained covered.

When she finally woke up, she looked rested and more cheerful. After I had dressed her I gave her a few teaspoonfuls of strained oatmeal (without milk). I was, of course, prepared for her to vomit again, but to my greatest joy and delight the food stayed in her stomach. It seems remarkable that something so simple as a vinegar compress could do such wonders. But it did, and she did not vomit again, nor did she have any more diarrhea. I continued giving her small quantities of the oatmeal every half hour, and in the evening added a little warm milk to it. To still her thirst I gave her the first day only plain water, almost lukewarm, and only one or two swallows at a time, though very often.

The following day I made her another compress as a precaution and started her gradually on her regular diet. By this time she was really hungry and with her increased appetite she was soon her normal self again.

If the first compress, complemented by a second one, had not helped so quickly, I should have repeated it every other day, if necessary for two weeks, until she was well again.

CASE No. 2: CHRONIC DIARRHEA

Under Case No. 1 I described how I treated acute diarrhea with a simple application. However, for chronic diarrhea more has to be done, and the following water applications should be used. If you put these to the test you will find that you get remarkable results if you follow directions exactly:

1. VINEGAR-WATER COMPRESS ON ABDOMEN:

One a day for two weeks, in the evening, every other day during third week if necessary (for details see Case No. 1 of this chapter) however under

PROCEDURE:

5. is repeated twice

2. HALF BATH:

Daily for two weeks, in the morning, twice a week during third week (for details see Chapter 6, 3, also Comments)

3A. UPPER SPONGING:

Daily for two weeks, in the afternoon, twice a week during third week (for details see Chapter 8, Case No. 1, also Comments)

or

3B. UPPER SPRAY:

Every other day for two weeks, in the afternoon, once a week during third week (for details see Chapter 11, 1, also Comments)

4. THREE HERB TEA MIXTURE:

One cupful every other day, taken one-third morning, noon and night, for three weeks, (for details see Chapter 39, 5, also Comments)

5. JUNIPER BERRIES (DRIED)

Four to eight berries eaten every other day alternating with the tea under 4.

Comments

The compress has a soothing and healing effect on the stomach and intestines. However, the half bath, upper sponging or spray not only improve and strengthen the stomach and intestines, but the entire system. The tea mixture and the juniper berries have their healing herbal effect on the stomach and intestines in improving the quantity and quality of digestive juices.

After three weeks there should be a marked improvement. To keep the system in proper functioning it is advisable to continue the half bath and upper sponging once a week.

18

Eliminating Gas Pains

As a young girl I used to suffer off and on from stomach gas pains. I had medical attention for this condition but without experiencing much improvement. However, since I have used the following water applications I have never suffered from gas pains:

1. COMPRESS ON THE ABDOMEN:

Every twelve to fifteen minutes, until pain is completely gone (for details see Chapter 17, Case No. 1, also Comments).

2. HIP SPRAY:

Two each week for three weeks, thereafter one every other week (for details see Chapter 7, Case No. 1, 1, also Comments).

3. HALF BATH:

Two each week for three weeks, thereafter one every other week (see TONSILLITIS, Chapter 6, 3, also Comments).

4. UPPER SPONGING:

One each week for three weeks, thereafter one every other week (for details see Chapter 8, Case No. 1, 3, also Comments).

5. UPPER SPRAY:

One each week for three weeks, thereafter one every other week, (for details see Chapter 11, 1, also Comments).

Comments on 1. Compress on Abdomen

With each compress, which I renewed every twelve to fifteen minutes, putting them on as warm as possible, the pain became less severe and my abdomen less distended until the gases finally did not bother me any further. Also my stomach felt light and clean; even my throat and head felt clearer.

Comments on 2. to 5. Cold Sprays and Baths

My whole system was strengthened, particularly my abdomen, which seemed to have contracted. The formation of new gases was prevented and all impurities seemed to have been cleared out.

19

Healing Pneumonia

When my little daughter was about two and a half years old she had pneumonia, with high fever and delirium. The doctor ordered lukewarm sponges and told me to keep her warm in bed. I was to give her only fruit juices and nothing else to eat. Although she was very sick, the doctor hesitated to send her to the hospital. He told me that I seemed to be a competent person and would be able to give her the best of care. To take the child away from me would mean to add the hurt of homesickness, which would tend to make her condition worse.

The first day the doctor was not able to detect the exact location of the inflammation, but on the second day he pointed out to me one area on her chest and one on her back. He told me then that it would take at least eight days before her condition would improve.

As soon as I knew the location of the inflammation, I made the following application:

1. PLASTER OF POT CHEESE (POULTICE):

One each day, for as many days as needed, for which I arranged the following

SUPPLIES:

1. one pound of pot cheese, plain, uncreamed, in lumps (not the cottage type),

2. a small bowl and wooden spoon
3. a strainer and glass of cold water,
4. four small pieces of kitchen towel, about six inches square each,
5. a bath towel folded twice into four layers, and followed this

PROCEDURE:

1. I pressed the pot cheese through the strainer into the bowl (with the wooden spoon),
2. added the cold water very gradually as I stirred the pot cheese until it had the consistency of a salve.
3. spread one-quarter of the quantity (with the spoon) on one of the four kitchen-towel squares, about half an inch thick, leaving about one inch dry margin all around,
4. rolled up my little girl's pajama top and immediately placed this plaster carefully on her chest, right on the area indicated by the doctor,
5. covered the plaster quickly with the folded bath towel, having the latter overlap the plaster all around by at least an inch,
6. rolled down her pajama top and covered her well with the regular bedding, up to her chin and over her shoulders, tucking it in well all around, and stayed with her at all times to make sure the plaster remained in place and that she was well covered,
7. after about ten minutes prepared the second plaster, the same as under 3., and checked the first plaster finding it to be warm and very dry, holding firmly together.
8. without uncovering my little girl too much, removed the dry plaster carefully and replaced it immediately with the second plaster, proceeding as under 5. and 6.,
9. about fifteen minutes after having put on the second plaster, prepared the third plaster, the same as under 3. and checked the second plaster (finding

it again warm and fairly dry, holding together in a somewhat looser way), replaced it immediately with the third plaster, proceeding as under 5. and 6.,

10. proceeded the same as under 9. for the fourth plaster,

11. after the fourth plaster had been in place for about twenty minutes, removed it together with the bath towel, rolled down the pajama top and replaced the bedding, staying with my little girl for another hour to make certain that she was covered and warm at all times,

12. repeated 1. to 11. the next day on the area of her back indicated by the doctor, for which purpose I put my little girl on her stomach.

2. FULL BATH:

(Fig. 20 shows you correct position)
One every morning during the first week, one every other day during the second week, for which I arranged the following

SUPPLIES:

1. the tub filled with the coldest water possible,
2. a large bath sheet spread out over the seat and back of the bathroom chair, made the following

PROVISIONS:

1. the bedroom and bathroom were warm,
2. there was no draft from any door or window,
3. my little girl felt warm, for which purpose I kept her covered in bed long enough so that she felt warm all over, and followed this

PROCEDURE:

1. I carried my little girl into the bathroom and re-moved her pajamas as fast as possible,
2. put my left arm around her back, holding her firmly under her left armpit, and with my right hand held her feet together around her ankles,

3. dipped her, feet first, into the cold water, gradually but reasonably fast submerging her whole body up to her neck, just one, two, three, and out again,

4. sat her on the bath sheet, which was spread out over the chair, quickly folded the corners over her shoulders and wrapped the rest of the bath sheet all around her,

5. carried her to bed without delay, covered her up to her neck and tucked in all around, especially behind her shoulders, staying with her to make sure that she remained covered at all times,

6. after an hour removed the bath sheet and put on her pajamas as quickly as possible, keeping her in bed during the first week, but dressing her warmly and letting her get up during the second week.

Comments on 1. Pot-Cheese Plaster

Before I put on the first plaster my little girl was delirious, but soon after the plaster was on her chest she became quiet and relaxed. The plaster must have had a soothing effect on her because after a few minutes she fell asleep.

When I removed the first plaster I found that it was almost like a shoe sole. I held it up between my thumb and forefinger on one corner to see whether it would come apart, but to my surprise it stayed in one piece and certainly did not look anything like the soft pot cheese spread I had put on the cloth. It was much darker in color—incredible. I had never experienced anything like it and could hardly believe it. I then realized that if the cottage cheese had changed its nature so drastically, it must have done so by the impurities it had drawn out of the body. I was convinced that the lungs had greatly benefited by it, although it was beyond my understanding how this simple method could do so much good.

The second plaster also came off in one piece, but I had to handle it more carefully since it was less firm. I was very glad to find it a little looser, since this proved to me that there were already fewer impurities in the body, even though the improvement was ever so slight. My little girl seemed to be breathing a little easier, and the temperature had gone down somewhat.

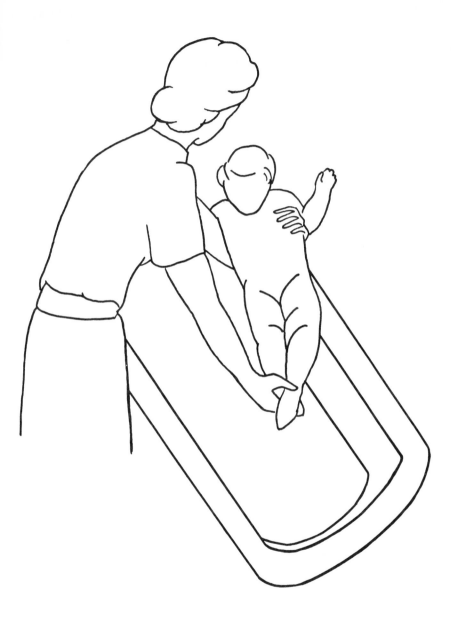

Figure 20: Position for placing child in Full Bath application for pneumonia.

Also the third plaster came off comparatively easily, again a shade looser so that it fell apart when I held it up. This meant to me another step forward in the healing process.

The fourth and final plaster was still soft when I took it off, and I had to be very careful to get every bit of pot cheese removed from the chest. I was inclined to accept this as proof that the plasters had healed the inflammation in this area entirely, and could hardly wait until the next morning to hear the doctor's opinion.

My little daughter had been sleeping most of the time and looked a little brighter when she woke up. She was also a little more willing to drink her fruit and vegetable juices. She still had some temperature, which I knew to be caused by the area in her back. But she had a much better night.

The next morning when the doctor examined her, he listened first with his stethoscope at the original area on her chest, then all over her chest, but always coming back to the original area. I could see that he was puzzled. Then he turned over and listened on her back, where he found the inflamed area immediately. He expressed his surprise that there was no more inflammation in front and stated that it had all concentrated now in the back. He rechecked the front again and shook his head: there was nothing there any more.

This simple remedy, outlined in the foregoing, had done wonders indeed. I collected myself enough to ask the doctor to indicate to me the inflamed back area. I could hardly wait for him to leave so that I could prepare for another series of pot-cheese plasters.

I put the plasters on the inflamed area in her back. I was glad that my little girl stayed put willingly on her stomach for the entire hour. She was, of course, still too weak to struggle against it. Also, I felt that she liked the plasters because they had a soothing effect.

With the four plasters I had similar experiences as the day before, a very good sign that they were doing a good job. After the last plaster had done its work, my little girl's temperature was almost normal, she was relaxed and looked more cheerful than she had done in a long time. She started to ask for her fruit juices and even ate a little oatmeal that evening. By all appearances her pneumonia was healed, and I could hardly wait for the next day to hear the doctor's opinion.

When he examined her, he was visibly amazed that he could not find a trace of the inflammation and could not comprehend it. He checked her over and over, front and back, and finally admitted that the pneumnonia had disappeared entirely. My joy was complete, and for the first time in many a day was I totally relieved.

I kept my little girl in bed for four more days until she was strong enough to get up gradually.

Comments on 2. Full Bath

When I dipped my little girl into the cold water she did not cry at all, but just caught her breath for a moment. And she never resisted being dipped into the water. She almost acted as if she welcomed the cold bath, apparently knowing how good it made her feel. As soon as I had tucked her in, she looked so relaxed and happy, and in the beginning she seemed to be glad to just lie quietly. But as she gradually improved she became restless so that I had to sing to her, show her pictures and toys, and play for her. At such times I also removed the bath sheet after half an hour and put on her nightgown, as quickly as possible, but kept her well covered for another half hour before I let her move around.

With each cold bath she improved visibly. Her appetite improved gradually and so did her color and her strength and vitality.

The cold baths became even more of a necessity when I found that her ears were discharging pus. (See Chapter 20, Case No. 1, EAR INFECTION.) By the time I had discovered the ear infection the cold baths apparently had already had some beneficial effect on the inner ears and had started to reduce the infection.

20

Taking Care of an Ear
Infection and
Earache

I happened to meet the sister of a famous physician and she was suffering at the time from an ear infection. I mentioned to her the beneficial effects of foot wrappings in water applications, expecting her to laugh at the idea. Instead she told me of her experience in Switzerland where she went to school. During that time she already had ear trouble, and the Swiss family with whom she lived suggested to her putting on wet socks with dry heavy woolen socks over them when going to bed at night. She followed their advice, and the next morning her earache was gone.

This is a very simple and effective way to get rid of an earache. It tends to draw the pressure away from the head and bring on a more balanced blood circulation, with the result that the ear improves also. If you should ever try it, you will find out how quickly you get healing help.

However, if the infection is more serious, then the following three cases will give you additional information, so that you may try the method best suited for you. While the case history concerns my daughter, you may easily adapt the application procedures for adult use.

CASE No. 1: EAR INFECTION

At the time my little daughter had pneumonia, she had also developed infected ears. She had never complained about any pain, probably because she was too sick with pneumonia, and by the time her pneumonia was better, her ears had also improved by the very applications I had used for the pneumonia. I had found out about the ear infection when I discovered one morning that her bedding was soiled with discharge on both sides of her head. When the doctor called that day I brought this to his attention. He subsequently examined her ears and found them both infected. He was very glad, though, that the infection had opened by then so that he did not have to puncture the inner ears. He advised me to rinse her ears with a lukewarm salt water solution, which I did the first day only. Instead I preferred to make the following applications:

1. EAR RINSE OF SCOURING RUSH:

(Latin: Equisetum arvense) (See Figure 21 showing position to be taken)
Once a day for seven days, for which I arranged the following

SUPPLIES:
1. one teaspoonful scouring rush tea,
2. one cup of boiling water,
3. a strainer and glass
4. a small syringe,
5. a pail
6. a towel
7. cotton, and followed this

PROCEDURE:
1. I poured the boiling water over the tea and let it steep for five to ten minutes until it had the right temperature of about 96°,
2. strained the tea into a glass and filled the syringe,
3. put the pail on the floor next to my chair and laid my little girl flat on her back in my lap with her head extended over the pail,

4. a. squeezed the syringe very gently into her right ear so that there was no air pressure and the herb tea almost just leaked into her ear, until about half the quantity was used, and then dried her ear with the towel,

   b. squeezed the rest of the tea, again gently, into her left ear, drying this also afterward,

5. put a little cotton in each ear just long enough to dry her ears on the inside,

6. thereafter kept the ears open so that the discharge could run out freely, but checked her ears frequently to see if I had to dab them dry with a little cotton.

2. FULL BATH:

One every day for one week, one every other day during second week (see PNEUMONIA, Chapter 19, 2).

Figure 21: Position for Ear Rinse of child.

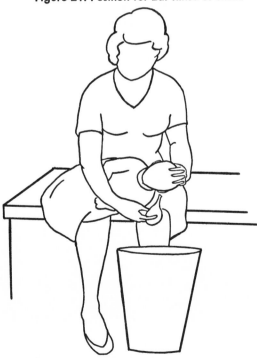

Comments on 1. Rinse of Scouring Rush

I knew from past experience that the scouring rush cleanses very thoroughly and at the same time has a very soothing effect. It heals beautifully and completely only after all impurities are cleaned out.

It is almost unbelievable, but every morning for three days I found the bedding of my little girl soaked with discharge from her ears. It was somewhat frightening. During the subsequent days, however, it became less every day until at the end of the week her ears had finally dried up. Because of my past experience with scouring rush I knew for certain that nothing had been left behind and that the ears were beautifully clean before they finally healed up.

Comments on 2. Full Bath

The cold full baths had taken the pressures away from her head and lessened the pain. The baths brought normal circulation all through the body, thereby hastening the healing of the ears, at the same time hardening and toughening the body and all organs. (This has been called the "total body concept" for healing.)

GENERAL

The healing was so perfect and complete and the ears became so healthy that now after twenty-eight years I can testify that my daughter's hearing is perfect. In all these years she has had an earache only once, namely in her teens after skiing on a very cold and windy day.

CASE No. 2: EAR INFLAMMATION

When my second daughter was seven months old she suffered from infected ears. She cried and whimpered almost continuously, turning her head from one side to the other. Since she was so small I did not dare to give her a cold full bath because I did not know whether children could be started that young. Therefore I called the doctor immediately and he diagnosed an ear infection, advising me to rinse the ears mornings and evenings with warm salt water and to keep the baby warm.

I followed his instructions very conscientiously, although the rinsings seemed to be rather painful for the baby. However, they did not seem to improve conditions sufficiently. The baby kept on crying the same as before. Only when I held her upright in my arms did she seem to feel a little better. Apparently the upright position diminished the pressure in her head. As soon as I held her level she cried again.

After having walked the floor with her for two nights I reasoned with myself that a cold bath would take the pressure away from her ears and relieve the pain, at the same time bringing proper circulation and healing. I finally convinced myself that if I proceeded with the utmost of care and accuracy, a cold bath could not do her any harm but only help her.

Therefore I proceeded to give her a

FULL BATH:

Two a day, with four hours' interval, for as many days as needed (see PNEUMONIA, Chapter 19, 2).

Comments

I did not remove the bath sheet as mentioned under Chapter 19, 2., 6. because she had fallen fast asleep. Instead I waited until she awoke, which was four hours later.

When I dipped my little girl into the cold water she did not cry at all, but just caught her breath for a moment, and when I had tucked her in warmly in bed she seemed very relaxed and apparently the pain had somewhat subsided, because she went to sleep almost immediately. I sat with her for an hour to make sure that she would not uncover herself. After the first hour I only checked from time to time.

I was greatly relieved that she slept so peacefully, and was surprised that she kept on sleeping and did not awake until four hours later. When she finally awoke the painful expression had left her face and she seemed to be much better. After I had given her some food and repeated the cold bath, the same as the first one, she again slept for four hours. To my greatest joy she awoke without crying. All pain seemed to have gone, which seemed almost incredible. She ate well and seemed very happy. Her temperature was normal, and from then on she resumed a normal life.

The earache did not return; neither did my daughter have any earache as a child or adolescent—I believe mainly because she walked barefoot at every opportunity, and whenever she had a cold I gave her a cold full bath immediately.

It may seem amazing to you how two cold baths of about a few seconds each have had such a marvelous result. However, the proof of healing with water applications in helping the body to help itself to vibrant health, at practically any age, speaks for itself!

CASE No. 3: EARACHE

We had gone skiing to the White Mountains with the children, staying in our ski cabin. My elder daughter had gone to the top of Cranmore Mountain on a day that was bitter cold and very windy. Apparently her knitted cap was not warm enough, so that she came home with an earache. Even in the warm cabin the earache did not get better, and it kept her from falling asleep at night.

If we had been at home I should have given her a cold

FULL BATH:

One every hour or every few hours, until pain relieved (see PNEUMONIA, Chapter 19, 2 or INSOMNIA, Chapter 10, 4), but since we did not have the usual bathroom facilities, I applied instead a

FOOT WRAPPING:

One at bedtime, on as many evenings as needed, (see WEAK ANKLES, Chapter 13, Case No. 4).

Comments on Foot Wrapping

After the wrappings had been on her feet for an hour, I dipped the kitchen towels again and applied them as before. Thereafter my daughter fell asleep. I had told her in advance that if she would fall asleep I should not want to remove the wrappings in order not to wake her, but leave them on for the night. However, as soon as she should wake up, either during the night or in the morning, she should remove the entire wrappings immediately and then keep her feet well covered for at least an hour, which she did.

She slept well through the night, and the next morning her earache was gone, which made her very happy because she did not have to miss any skiing. That day was a little warmer and less windy so that she enjoyed her skiing thoroughly. Her ears never bothered her again.

21

It Was Easy to Get
Rid of My Appendicitis

I had a mild attack of appendicitis while I was pregnant. I did not want to call the doctor before having tried a cold compress. However, I was hesitant to apply ice-cold water, not knowing whether it was safe during pregnancy. Therefore I decided to make a pot-cheese plaster instead.

A short time after the baby was born I had another attack. My obstetrician diagnosed it as appendicitis and told me to apply ice packs, at the same time observing a liquid diet. As much as I favor ice-cold water, I feel that ice itself is too drastic and should not touch the body. Therefore I decided to make a cold compress.

In order to prevent any recurrence I also started taking hip sprays. In other words, I took the following applications for appendicitis:

1A. POT-CHEESE PLASTER ON RIGHT SIDE OF ABDOMEN:

One hour each day, for as many days as needed (see PNEUMONIA, Chapter 19, 1).

1B. COMPRESS ON RIGHT SIDE OF ABDOMEN:

One hour each day, for as many days as needed (see COUGH, Chapter 3).

2. HIP SPRAY:

One a day for one week, thereafter once a week (for details see Chapter 7, Case No. 1, 1).

Comments on 1A. Pot-Cheese Plaster

With each plaster the pain became a little less, and after an hour it was so slight that I did not want to bother the doctor about it. The next day the pain was gone entirely. I assume that the short half baths I had taken all through my pregnancy had also prevented the appendicitis from becoming severe.

Comments on 1B. Compress

The ice-cold water was very soothing and it numbed the pain, which became less with each new dipping so that there was finally only a little soreness left. The next day I repeated the compress for another hour and soon the pain was gone.

Comments on 2. Hip Spray

While spraying the front of my right leg I held the hose each time for a few seconds on the area of the appendix. These sprays tended to have regulated the circulation not only of the blood but also the bowels, and all impurities must have been carried away, because I have not had another attack since. (See also COMMENTS ON HIP SPRAY, Chapter 7, Case No. 1, 1.)

22

Relieving and Stopping
a Toothache

While on a trip, I started getting a toothache, which upset me because I could not go to our dentist in New York for the next two days, and I did not want to go to a strange dentist. I tried to relieve the ache by taking aspirin, but it did not help enough. When I could not stand the pain any longer I used cold water and applied the following:

1. KNEE SPRAY:

Two a day, for as many days as needed (see MUCUS, Chapter 11, 2).

2. CHEEK SPRAY:

Four a day, for as many days as needed, for which I arranged the following

SUPPLIES:

1. a rubber hose (or handspray without the spray head) attached to the bathtub faucet,
2. a bath towel draped over my shoulder to keep myself from getting wet,
3. a face towel (in readiness),
   and followed this

PROCEDURE:

1. I held my cheek over the bathtub and sprayed it with the coldest water possible by going up and down from the jaw to the eye in even strokes, holding the hose about three inches away from the cheek, for about twenty seconds or as long as I could stand it,
2. without drying my face held the face towel, folded double, against my cheek until it felt normal, i.e., for about half an hour,
3. repeated the sprays as soon as the pain came back, taking four sprays in all the first day, and two the second.

Comments on 1. Knee Spray

It seemed to me as if the knee spray had drawn the blood from my head. My feet felt warm soon afterward, while my head felt light, with the pressure considerably relieved and the toothache somewhat diminished.

Comments on 2. Cheek Spray

Soon after I had started spraying, the pain stopped; however, I continued as long as I could stand the cold water because I wanted to have a long-lasting result. After about two hours the pain came back, and as soon as I started spraying again, it stopped. Thereafter the intervals became longer so that I had to spray only twice during the night.

The next day the pain was rather bearable, and I took two more sprays, and the following day I went to my regular dentist to have the tooth filled.

I have not had any severe toothache since that time which I attribute mainly to the cold-water sprays and baths I take regularly. I have had cavities filled, but I have not lost a single tooth since childhood. My gums are firm and healthy.

23

Stopping Influenza
(Grippe)

At one time I had a severe case of influenza, with the usual symptoms, including a high temperature. I immediately started taking the following steps:

1. FULL SPONGING:

One every hour for eight hours during the first day, one every hour for four hours during the second day, one in the morning and one at night for the next two days, (see HEAD COLD, Chapter 2, Case No. 1).

2. WATER-WITH-LEMON DRINKS:

Six glasses the first day at two or three hours interval (without eating any food), thereafter one glass half an hour before each meal for as many days as needed, for which I used the following

PREPARATION:

1. I squeezed the juice of half a lemon, well strained, into a drinking glass,
2. added enough cold water to fill the glass,
3. stirred well, without using any sugar or other sweetening.

Comments on 1. Full Sponging

Before I started the spongings my skin felt very hot and dry, but already after the first sponging it started to get gradually damp. Soon after the third sponging I actually started to perspire. My skin never got hot and dry again. I repeated the spongings every hour, although I was wet with perspiration.

After each sponging I felt very refreshed and perked right up, my head felt lighter and the headache was gone. However, after about forty or fifty minutes I was really looking forward to the next cold sponging because I began to feel somewhat miserable again, but this feeling became less after each sponging.

After eight spongings the perspiration had almost stopped, and I got up after having rested another hour. By that time it was evening and I prepared dinner for my family, although I felt somewhat weak, but my headache was gone and I began to feel hungry. I had some soup and after a while felt a normal sleepiness and went to bed again. I slept well through the night and awoke light and refreshed. I took four more spongings after a light breakfast and got up for lunch. Thereafter I attended to my usual duties as a housewife, although I still felt a little weak. However, I was very hungry and ate well. The two cold spongings during the next few days seemed just right for me to improve my health and strength, and after a week I was my old self again.

It was incredible to me that the cold water had cured me of the influenza so quickly that I was able to get up the next day, while in former years it had taken about two weeks before I could go back to work, and before my appetite returned to normal.

24

Making a Ganglion
(Node) Disappear

During a game of tennis, a fast ball hit me very hard on my underarm about half way between my wrist and elbow. It was very painful, and after a few days I noticed a small knot forming at the very spot, alongside my bone. The knot finally grew to the size of a small marble. It was hard, but it did not hurt, not even when I wiggled it around. I had it for a number of years, but did not pay any attention to it.

In order to get rid of this unsightly swelling, I started to take regularly a cold

ARM SPRAY:

(Figures 22 and 23 following will guide you in its application) Four or five times a week, during every week whenever possible, for which I arranged the following

SUPPLIES:

1. a rubber hose, or a handspray (with the sprayhead removed), attached to the bathtub faucet,
2. a bath towel,
   and followed this

PROCEDURE:

1. I removed my pajama top, wrapped a large bath towel around my chest under the armpits, and bent over the bath tub,

2. with the coldest water possible, started to spray my right hand at No. 1 and proceeded slowly to No. 2., holding the hose about three inches away from my arm in such a way that the water would cover the whole arm like a sheet (never running in trickles), waited at No. 2 for a few moments and then returned to No. 1, repeating the same routine up to five times,

3. started to spray my left hand at No. 3 and proceeded, the same as for the right arm, to No. 4 and back again to No. 3, also five times,

4. without drying myself placed the bath towel over my shoulders like a cape and went to bed until I felt warm and dry, or—on hot days—dressed and moved around until my arms were dry.

Comments

I kept these sprays up regularly and am still applying them now, because they are so refreshing and toughened my arms so that I can wear sleeveless dresses all through the year without feeling cold.

I had entirely forgotten the ganglion until one day I wanted to find out whether it was getting smaller, and was puzzled for a moment when I could not find it. I thought I had by mistake felt the wrong arm, but it was not on the other arm either. It was simply gone!

You may doubt that something so hard and lasting as a node or knot on the flesh could be made to disappear just by running cold water over it. But there was no remaining sign of it. I could not even find the spot where it had been, and no scar whatever existed. In general, the careful armspray clearly improves my blood circulation and helps to keep it normal. It can also be beneficial for rheumatism and arthritis. Many seeming miracles can be performed by the body itself if only you assist good circulation of the blood and body fluids.

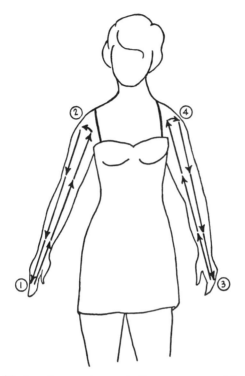

Figure 22: Arm Spray—Arrows indicate patterns of flow of spray.

Although the armspray takes the pressure away from the heart by drawing the blood into the hands, persons with heart trouble should first start walking barefoot for a while, then walk in cold water for a few days (for details see Chapter 13, Case No. 1) and finally start with short knee and arm sprays, increasing them gradually (for details on knee spray, see Chapter 11, 2). The good results in improving the heart and strengthening the entire body will speak for themselves. Good circulation means good health for the total body.

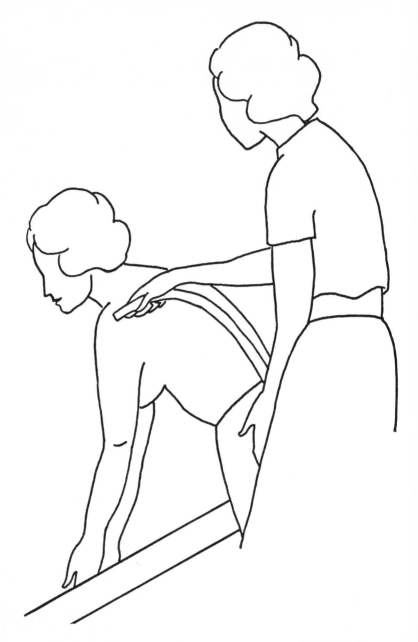

Figure 23: Position for giving Arm Spray. (See also Figure 22)

25

Contagious Diseases

At the slightest sign of indisposition or temperature in our family we apply cold water immediately, even if we don't know the cause of the illness.

A full sponging or full bath is always beneficial. It may not attack the source of the illness directly, but it is an overall help in improving conditions for the entire body and in reducing the temperature. In severe illnesses the fever will return soon and often; however it will finally be conquered by repeated applications.

The three cases which follow will tell you about the successes we have had and guide you in your need for you and your family, so that you, too, may be helped.

CASE No. 1: MEASLES

During one summer vacation we went to our ski cabin in the White Mountains. We had hardly arrived when my elder daughter came down with a fever, accompanied by a dry cough and watery eyes, and the younger one did the same, one day later.

If we had been at home, I should have given them the following applications:

1. FULL BATH:

Every hour for eight hours, or until temperature normal (see PNEUMONIA, Chapter 19, 2, or INSOMNIA, Chapter 10, 4).

2. HALF BATH:

Starting second day (after fever is down) daily for one week, (see TONSILLITIS, Chapter 6, 3).

3. SHORT WRAPPING:

One the third day, one the sixth day (for details see Chapter 8, Case No. 1, 5), but since we did not have the usual bathroom facilities, they took instead the following:

1A. FULL SPONGING:

Every hour for eight hours, or until temperature is normal, for which I arranged the following

SUPPLIES:

1. a bowl with ice-cold water,
2. a good-size facecloth,
3. a small bedsheet (instead of a bath sheet)
4. a bath towel
   and followed this

PROCEDURE:

1. I folded the bedsheet in half (bringing the top to the bottom) and layed it crosswise on the bed so that it would reach from the armpits to the legs,
2. placed the bath towel about half way above the bedsheet to reach from the neck to the elbow,
3. had my daughter undress completely and lie on her stomach on the towel and folded bedsheet,
4. dipped the face cloth into the cold water, squeezed out the excess water and as quickly as possible washed her back in even strokes, beginning at the shoulders and neck (including back of arms) and going all the way down to the heels, dipping the cloth frequently,
5. after having turned her over on her back, without drying her, proceeded in the same manner in front from the neck and shoulders (including the front of arms) all the way down to the toes,

6. without drying her, wrapped the folded bedsheet around her, tucking it in well, and folded the bath towel around her shouders like a cape, covering her well with sufficient blankets,

7. after an hour repeated 4. to 6.,

8. repeated 7. six times (eight sponges in all),

9. one hour after last sponging put on her pajamas with a sweater over the top for extra warmth and had her sit up in bed.

2A. QUICK DIP IN BROOK:

starting second day (after fever is down), daily for one week whenever weather is warm and sunny.

Comments

The morning after the full spongings they both were ready to get up. They looked and acted normal. The fever did not return. Soon red spots appeared, at first in their faces and then over their entire bodies. However they both ate and slept well, and within a few days the spots had disappeared.

It may seem incredible to you how both these girls recovered so quickly without any bad after-effects and without feeling sick for more than a few hours, when you think of how you may have suffered with measles during your childhood; how long you had to remain in bed and how extremely weak you felt when you finally got up.

The knowledge to apply the cold-water benefits properly may be able to spare your children an unnecessary prolonged illness.

CASE No. 2: CHICKEN POX

One year our two daughters had a contagious disease as soon as we arrived at our summer home. This time it was chicken pox. Although their temperature was almost normal, I felt that it would be good to generally improve their blood circulation by a cold-water application.

If we had been at home I should have given them a cold

FULL BATH:

One in the morning and one at night, for three days (see PNEUMONIA, Chapter 19, 2, or INSOMNIA, Chapter 10, 4), but since we did not have the usual bath facilities, they took instead a cold

FULL SPONGING:

One in the morning and one at night for three days (for details see Case No. 1, 1A).

Comments on Cold Full Bath

I always prefer a cold full bath to a cold sponging because it goes faster, therefore the body itself does not cool off so much, and the blood reaction toward fighting off the cold water is faster, bringing about a quicker stimulation and warming effect. According to my experience the all-over improvement is much faster. Also, the children prefer a cold bath, because they get it over with much quicker and find themselves back in bed and getting warmer much faster, with the result that they also feel better sooner.

Comments on Full Sponging

The cold spongings seemed to take the heat and itching out of the pox. Those which they had scratched open healed very quickly and the others disappeared soon.

The children kept up their regular activities. Their appetite remained good throughout, and they slept soundly.

CASE No. 3: GERMAN MEASLES (RUBELLA)

When German measles struck our children, at first I did not know what was wrong with them when they asked me for a cold bath because they were not feeling well. It may sound incredible that a child should ask to be put into a tub of ice-cold water, but since my children knew from experience that one second in cold water makes them feel so much better, it was only natural for them to ask.

Therefore I gave them a cold

FULL BATH:

Once a day until the marks had disappeared (see INSOM-NIA, Chapter 10, 4). If the children had felt too sick to get up, I should have given them instead a cold

FULL SPONGING:

Three or four times a day until the marks had disappeared (for details see Case No. 1, 1A).

Comments on Full Bath

As usual, both felt much better after each cold full bath. Soon after the first bath the marks appeared. They were less severe than those of regular measles and also disappeared sooner.

Since the taking of cold full baths is a cleansing process, we kept them up until the marks were entirely gone, although it would not have been necessary to keep them up that long just to combat the illness. But with the additional baths the children recovered unusually fast and were soon full of energy and vitality.

Comments on Full Sponging

Whenever my children felt too weak or too sick to get up, I always found it advisable and very helpful to give them cold spongings first until they felt better, and then follow these up with cold full baths.

The cold spongings not only normalize the temperature in the body, but are also very refreshing and prevent headcolds. They improve the appetite and seem to make the skin breath properly and normally.

26

Overcoming Depression

When my elder daughter was in high school she experienced a period of depression, during which she cried at the slightest provocation. She stayed alone in her room and did not want to talk to anyone. She even kept the door to her room closed, which was very unusual. If I succeeded in talking to her with the intention of cheering her, she would only start crying. She could not explain her depression to me. She only knew that a terrible fear had gotten hold of her. She was not physically ill, although she ate very little. She had lost all interest in the things she usually enjoyed.

I wanted to help her, and finally suggested to her the following series of cold-water applications:

1. FULL SPONGING:

Twice daily for seven days with half water and half vinegar (for details see Chapter 2, Case No. 1, also Comments).

2. HALF BATH:

On Monday, Wednesday, and Friday during second, third, and fourth week (see TONSILLITIS, Chapter 6, 3).

3. UPPER SPONGING:

On Tuesday, Thursday, and Saturday during second week (for details see Chapter 8, Case No. 1, also Comments).

4. SHORT WRAPPING:

On Sunday during second, third, and fourth week (for details see Chapter 8, Case No. 1, also Comments).

5. FULL BATH:

One a week, starting fifth week for as many weeks as desired (see INSOMNIA, Chapter 10, 4). She was willing to take only the FULL BATH, which we started immediately, once a day for seven days.

Comments on Full Bath

It seemed that the cold full bath regulated her blood circulation, thereby restoring the natural body warmth and the proper working of the entire system.

After each cold bath my daughter looked very relaxed and for a short time afterward seemed to be very much at ease, as if she had experienced a great relief.

From day to day she improved steadily, and at the end of the week was cheerful and her old self again. I was happy and grateful at the quick, good results of the cold full bath, so that none of the other applications outlined were necessary.

My daughter has always been in good health and good spirits since that time, which is now more than fifteen years ago.

27

Getting Rid of Sciatica

During one year I did a lot of gardening. One day I had a sharp pain in my right thigh. I tried to ignore it and continued with my garden work, since I did not suspect that this pain was caused by strain. From day to day the pain became more severe, until finally it was so bad that it kept me from sleeping. Also walking was painful. I commuted to and from work in New York. Although the seats on the train were upholstered, I could feel every movement of the train, and sitting down and getting up was a very slow process. I had to hold on to the seat in front of me and let myself down slowly into the seat. On arrival I pulled myself slowly up out of the seat. By that time I had had to discontinue all garden work. Days went by, but the pain did not diminish.

I prepared to take the following series of applications:

1. BACK SPRAY:

Every morning for two weeks (see CONSTIPATION, Chapter 12, 3).

2. UPPER SPRAY:

Every other evening (Monday, Wednesday, Friday) for two weeks (see MUCUS, Chapter 11, 1).

3. HALF BATH:

Every other evening (Tuesday, Thursday, Saturday) for two weeks (see TONSILLITIS, Chapter 6, 3).

4. HIP SPRAY:

Every other day during third and fourth week (for details see Chapter 7, Case No. 1, also Comments).

Comments on Hip Spray

I began with the hip spray first, planning to use the other applications only if the hip spray alone were not successful.

When spraying my right leg the first evening, I held the hose on the painful area as long as I could stand it. At first the pain seemed even greater than before; nevertheless I continued holding the cold water on this spot until there was a certain numbness and the pain was just a dull feeling. After the spray I stayed in bed for an hour. At first my leg felt very warm and comfortable; the pain had eased considerably, but gradually it seemed to increase again. Therefore I repeated the spray after one hour, again holding the cold water on the painful spot until the pain was gone. When I was back in bed my leg felt much better and I went to sleep soon afterward.

When I awoke in the morning, having slept all through the night, I found that I could move about much better. Toward evening the pain had increased somewhat, and I therefore repeated the sprays, again two, as the day before. After three days and six sprays the pain was gone entirely.

Although I have been doing rather strenuous garden work during the past few years, I have not had sciatica again. I assume that the cold-water sprays helped so quickly because I applied them comparatively soon after the onset of the pain and also because I have been taking cold-water applications generally, thereby improving my overall physical condition. As has been truly said "An ounce of prevention is worth more than a pound of cure."

28

Getting Rid of Rheumatism

One winter I developed a very painful case of rheumatism in my right wrist. Because I had been taking arm sprays regularly I did not expect anything of this sort, and had been rather careless about drying my hands and wrists. Also, I had been wearing a gold bracelet on my right wrist constantly without ever removing it, even when taking a bath or spray. Often it was left wet and felt rather uncomfortable, but I paid little attention to it and let it get dry by itself. Because of this neglect a pain developed in my wrist, and finally became so severe that I had to do something about it. I therefore programmed the following two applications:

1. HAND SPRAY:

One every hour as often as pain returns for which I arranged the following

SUPPLIES:

1. a rubber hose or handspray (without the spray head) attached to the bathtub faucet,
2. a face towel and piece of string, and followed this

PROCEDURE:

1. I bent over the bathtub and sprayed the lower part of my underarm with the coldest possible water by

holding the hose about three inches away so that the water would cover my entire wrist like a sheet and run down my hand, keeping the hose thus in place until the pain stopped,

2. without drying my wrist and lower arm, wrapped them at once in the dry face towel, and tied it up with the string,

3. after half an hour removed the towel, but kept the hand active and warm.

2. HAND WRAPPING:

(Figure 24 following shows you its correct application)
Every evening as many evenings as necessary with the following

PREPARATIONS:

1. One tablespoonful of hay flowers to three cups of boiling water, letting it steep for five to ten minutes,

2. a small kitchen towel folded into four layers,

3. a face towel, and this

PROCEDURE:

1. The folded kitchen towel dipped into the warm herb tea (which may be strained), wrung out carefully (not too dry but not dripping wet) and wound around the wrist and hand in a very thorough manner so that the towel clings to the wrist all around, but not too tight in order not to hinder the blood circulation,

2. the dry face towel wound around the wet towel, overlapping well on both sides so that no draft can enter,

3. after one hour compress dipped into solution again and applied as under 1. and 2., for another hour,

4. after second hour the wet towel removed, a scarf wound loosely around the wrist for about thirty minutes to keep it warm.

Dispelling Rheumatism in Other Parts of the Body

If I had had rheumatism in other parts of my body, which I believe would have indicated that my system had to be cleared of impurities, I should have taken the following applications:

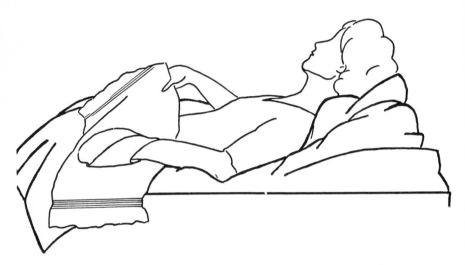

Figure 24: Position in resting with Hand Wrapping application for rheumatism.

1. SHORT WRAPPING:

Twice during first and second week, once a week during third to fifth week (for details see Chapter 40).

2. FULL SPONGING:

Once or twice daily for one week (for details see Chapter 2, Case No. 1).

3. HAY-FLOWER COMPRESS ON AFFECTED PART(S):

Once or twice daily for one week (for details see Chapter 8, Case No. 1, 4) (see also HAND WRAPPING, this chapter).

4. KNEE SPRAY:

One or twice daily and whenever pain returns for one week (for details see Chapter 11, 2, also Comments) holding hose on painful area until pain gone.

5. UPPER SPRAY:

Once or twice daily and whenever pain returns during first week, twice a week during second and third week, once a week during fourth and fifth week, (see MUCUS, Chapter 11, 1) holding hose on painful area until pain gone.

6. HIP SPRAY:

Twice a week during second and third week, once a week during fourth and fifth week (for details see Chapter 7, Case No. 1, 1, also Comments).

Comments on Hand Spray

In spite of the fact that the rheumatism had been brought about by wetness, I decided to use the cold-water spray and the hand wrapping. However, instead of starting with the latter, I tried the hand spray first, figuring that since the rheumatism attack was rather recent, I should get immediate results, which I certainly did.

At first the cold water was very painful, but I kept on spraying. Soon my wrist and hand became numb and the pain gradually less; however, I did not stop spraying until the pain was gone entirely.

After I had wrapped my hand and wrist in the face towel, a nice warmth developed and my wrist felt relaxed. After half an hour I went about my activities as usual and did not have any pain for about three hours.

When the pain returned I repeated the same procedure. This time the pain stayed away for a longer period and I repeated the spray only once more that same day and once the following morning. Thereafter the pain did not return, and I did not have to apply the hand wrapping at all.

I assume that the cold-water sprays helped so quickly because I applied them soon after the onset of the pain, and also because I have been taking arm sprays regularly, thereby bringing good circulation in my arms so that a simple local spray corrected the ailment.

29

Reducing Fever

Whenever any member of our family had a fever, I applied immediately one of the following:

1. FULL BATH:

Once every hour until fever stopped, one in the morning and evening of next day (see a. PNEUMONIA, Chapter 19, 2 for small children, and b. INSOMNIA, Chapter 10, 4 for adults).

2. FULL SPONGING:

Once every hour until fever stopped, one in the morning and evening of next day (for details and comments see a. Chapter 25, Case No. 1, for small children, and b. Chapter 2, Case No. 1 for adults).

Comments

Although at the start of a fever the cause of it is often not yet known, I always apply cold water immediately, since it cannot do any harm, no matter what illness has brought about the fever, but can only be beneficial.

In most cases immediately after the cold water was applied the temperature went back to normal for a while, then started to rise again gradually. However, after each additional application the temperature stayed normal longer, until finally it remained normal.

Our children were quite aware of the beneficial effects of cold water, so that whenever they had a fever, sometimes before I even was aware of it, they asked me to give them a cold bath. Ordinarily they shunned cold water, as most children do, but when they felt miserable with a fever it seemed natural for them to say: "Mother, I want a cold bath," because they knew that a cold bath would bring them quick relief and make them feel better. In that respect my children were not exceptional, because lately even my grandchildren have asked their mother for a cold bath when they did not feel well. Yes, water is the answer.

30

Obesity Need Not
Be a Problem

In spite of the fact that my mother and also my two grand-mothers were rather stout, my weight stayed normal all through the years. I firmly believe that the various cold-water applications have kept me from gaining weight. However, if obesity became a problem for me, then I should resolve to take the following:

1. HIP SPRAY:

One every morning for two weeks, one every other morning during third and fourth week, once a week thereafter until weight is normal (for details see Chapter 7, Case No. 1).

2. BACK SPRAY:

One every afternoon for two weeks, one every other after-noon during third and fourth week, once a week thereafter until weight is normal (see CONSTIPATION, Chapter 12, 3).

3. SHORT WRAPPING:

One every other evening for two weeks, twice a week during third and fourth week, once a week thereafter until weight is normal (for details see Chapter 40).

Comments

I have taken these applications at different times for various ailments and have continued the hip spray regularly once a week, together with knee and arm sprays four or five times a week (see Chapter 11, 2, and Chapter 5, Case No. 1, 1).

All of these have apparently improved my blood circulation, and the proper functioning of my glands was established thereby. I have a healthy appetite at all times, eat well-balanced meals and never had to go on a special diet. At the present printing of this book, I am sixty-three. I still wear the same size clothes I did when I was twenty-one.

I found that particularly the hip and back sprays were very envigorating and strengthened my body, while the short wrapping seemed to cleanse the whole system, including the vital organs, so that all impurities were discarded through the kidneys and bowels, noticeably at the time of the applications. Also, the water in the cells making up the body tended to be kept at a normal level with the water applications described in this book.

31

Getting Rid of Varicose Veins
in a Natural Way

I firmly believe that I have never had any varicose veins, not even during pregnancy, because I have taken cold-water applications regularly for more than thirty years. However, should they ever appear and be a problem to me then I should take the following applications:

1. HALF BATH:

Two mornings a week during first three weeks, one morning a week during second three weeks (see TONSILLITIS, Chapter 6, 3).

2. HIP SPRAY:

Four afternoons a week during first three weeks, one afternoon a week during second three weeks (for details see Chapter 7, Case No. 1, 1, also Comments).

3. BACK SPRAY:

Two mornings a week during first three weeks, one morning a week during second three weeks (see CONSTIPATION, Chapter 12, 3).

4. LEG WRAPPING:

(Figure 25 following shows you its correct application.)
Two nights a week during first three weeks, one night a week
thereafter as long as needed.

PREPARATIONS:

For one leg (double quantities to be used for both legs),
1. two cups of boiling water added to two teaspoonfuls
   of hay flowers, letting it steep for five to ten minutes,
2. two kitchen towels folded in half to fit from the knee
   to the ankle,
3. a bath towel,
4. a piece of plastic material to reach from the knee
   to the ankle.

PROCEDURE:

1. The plastic material put on the bed, (underneath the
   calf) and on top, the bath towel.
2. the kitchen towels dipped folded together into the
   warm herb tea (which may be strained), wrung out
   carefully, not too dry but not dripping wet, and
   wound around the calf to reach from the knee to the
   ankle, not too tight but close enough that the towels
   cling to the leg all around,
3. bath towel wound around the leg, closing off the wet
   kitchen towels around the knee and ankle, followed
   by the plastic material and then the usual bed covers.

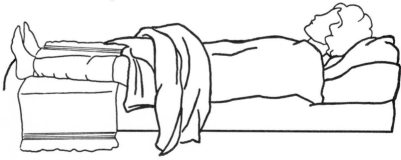

Figure 25: Positioning and detail of Leg Wrapping.

4. all wrappings removed after about one and a half hours, unless one has fallen asleep, in which case wrappings removed after awakening, but half an hour before getting up.

Comments on 4. Leg Wrapping

I have found when taking a leg wrapping that I can sleep beautifully and very soundly. This wrapping tends to improve the hearing and is very good for healing ear trouble in general. It serves to clean out internal body impurities, thereby improving the functioning of the veins in the interests of good circulation.

Comments on 1. 2. and 3. Applications

I have taken these applications at various times for other ailments and continued the half bath and hip spray regularly, together with knee and arm sprays (see Chapter 11, 2, and Chapter 5, Case No. 1, 1). All of these applications have cast their individual beneficial effects on legs, and particularly leg veins.

32

Help for Annoying
Headaches

As a young girl and also in my twenties I suffered greatly with headaches. But this evil burden disappeared soon after I had started using cold-water applications regularly. If I should ever be bothered with headaches again, I would make the following applications:

1. HALF BATH:

Monday, Wednesday, Friday morning for three weeks, once a week thereafter (see TONSILLITIS, Chapter 6, 3).

2. KNEE SPRAY:

Tuesday, Thursday, Saturday morning for three weeks, four or five times a week thereafter (see MUCUS, Chapter 11, 2).

3. UPPER SPRAY:

Tuesday, Thursday, Saturday afternoon for three weeks, occasionally thereafter, (see MUCUS, Chapter 11, 1).

4. SHORT WRAPPING:

Sunday and Wednesday afternoon for three weeks, occasionally thereafter (for details see Chapter 40).

5. WALKING BAREFOOT:

Daily whenever possible (for details see Chapter 13, Case No. 1, 2, also Comments).

Comments

I have taken these applications at various times for other ailments and have continued the half bath, knee spray and walking barefoot regularly, together with arm sprays (see Chapter 5, Case No. 1, 1).

All of these applications demonstrated their beneficial effects conclusively. My headaches disappeared, my mood became a happier one, my appetite and digestion were normalized and I slept soundly. Furthermore, my feet were always normally warm. I did not feel cold so easily and was also less susceptible to catching colds.

33

A Healthy Hair
Growth

I have always had a very healthy growth of hair, and even at age sixty-three my hair is as full and heavy as it was in my youth. I strongly believe that this is definitely the result of using some or all of the following applications regularly; or frequently:

1. HALF BATH:

Once or twice a week (see TONSILLITIS, Chapter 6, 3).

2. UPPER SPONGING:

Two or three times a week (for details see Chapter 8, Case No. 1, 3, also Comments).

3. KNEE SPRAY:

Four or five times a week (see MUCUS, Chapter 11, 2).

4. HEAD SPRAY:

(Figure 26 following will guide you in its correct application) Once a week, for which I arranged the following

SUPPLIES:

1. a rubber hose (or handspray without the spray head) attached to the bathtub faucet,

2. a bath towel,
   and followed this

PROCEDURE:

1. I bent over the bathtub and with the coldest water possible, holding the hose about three inches away from my head, started spraying behind my right ear, going alongside the neck to behind the left ear, then alongside the forehead back to behind the right ear, continuing in a spiral toward the center of the hair and letting the water run like a sheet over the whole head, never holding the hose long in one spot,

2. repeated this procedure up to five times, depending on how cold the water was and how long I could stand it,

3. dried my hair as thoroughly as possible with the bath towel by rubbing it and massaging the scalp lightly, using a dryer afterward.

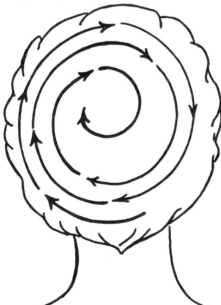

Figure 26: Head Spray—Arrows indicate pattern and direction of spray on the head.

Comments

This spray is very refreshing; the whole scalp seems to be tingling and alive, and the head feels warm and comfortable soon afterward. It is also beneficial for the eyes and ears, and has been reported to be effective in healing earache.

34

Improving the Functioning
of Glands

Because in our immediate family we have taken cold water applications regularly, or at least from time to time, we never had any symptoms of swollen glands, with one exception, in which case we used the applications given under Case No. 2 of this chapter, GLANDS IN GENERAL.

If you take a weekly half bath or hip spray and an upper sponging or upper spray you will keep a proper blood circulation in your system and thereby a normal functioning of all organs, including the glands. You will find that you have no serious problem with regard to any malfunctioning of glands. However, should you be in need of immediate help, you may find it in the applications given under the following two cases.

CASE No. 1: HOW A SERIOUS THYMUS CONDITION WAS HEALED

When D., the son of my younger daughter, was two months old, she took him for a checkup. The doctor listened on the boy's back to his breathing, listened to his crying and then saw him turn blue when he lay on his back. She thereupon informed my daughter that D. had to go into the hospital because of the danger of suffocation. There he was put under a tent and supplied with a mixture of oxygen and steam to help him breathe. A specialist was called in and confirmed the diagnosis of an enlarged thymus gland. When the pediatrician decided on X-ray treatments, my daughter and her husband went to the hospital and took the baby home. My daughter started the following applications immediately:

1. COMPRESS ON THYMUS:

All evening of the first day, all day long during the second day, with interruptions for feeding, etc. (same as COMPRESS ON CHEST, see COUGH, Chapter 3).

2. FULL BATH:

One every day for one week beginning on the third day, once a week thereafter for six months (see PNEUMONIA, chapter 19, 2).

Comments on Compress

The ice-water compress was put on the lower part of the throat, where the thymus is located. My daughter applied the compress almost constantly, whereas a maximum of two hours is more advisable. However, her success in overcoming the gland condition speaks for itself.

Comments on Full Baths

The cold FULL BATHS had been applied by my daughter for about seven months. These cold baths have developed D. into a very healthy and strong boy who is eight years old now and has never needed medical attention again.

CASE No. 2: GLANDS IN GENERAL

1. COMPRESS ON GLANDS:

Once a day for one to two hours, for as many days as needed (for details see Chapter 3).

2. HALF BATH:

One a day during first week, in the morning, one every other day during second week, twice a week during third and fourth week, once a week thereafter (for details see Chapter 6, 3, also Comments).

3A. UPPER SPONGING:

One a day during first week, in the afternoon, thereafter as often as half baths are taken, (for details see Chapter 8, Case No. 1, 3, also Comments). Or

3B. UPPER SPRAY:

One every other day during first week, afternoons, twice a week during second and third week, once a week thereafter, (for details see Chapter 11, 1, also Comments).

Comments on Compress

Whenever I have applied a compress for whatever purpose, I found that it had a most beneficial effect. It loosens, softens, dissolves, reduces and often seems to melt away any disorder. When removing the wet cloth you will find that it looks discolored, and when dipping it in the water that the latter becomes cloudy, a sign that the compress has drawn impurities out of the body through the pores.

Comments on Half Bath

You will find that the half bath improves the blood circulation considerably, thereby clearing any form of congestion, swelling, or inflammation, not only in the lower but also the upper part of the body. It is strengthening, develops a normal warmth all through the body, has a calming influence and helps to restore the body to good health.

Comments on Upper Sponging/Upper Spray

The upper spray has a much stronger effect than the upper sponging. For weak persons or those with a heart or lung ailment, it is therefore necessary to start with the sponging, and after a few days with a very light upper spray, which may then be gradually increased from day to day. The upper spray should always be taken in connection with a knee spray, hip spray, or half bath.

You will note that after the upper spray a pleasant warmth develops. It seems to loosen all impurities and to clean them out thoroughly. Together with the hip spray or half bath, it regulates the blood circulation and induces the entire system, including glands, to function properly. The upper sponging is milder and therefore its effect also slower, but essentially the same.

35

Excessive Perspirations

Very often the cause for excessive perspiration, whether of the feet or any other part of the body, lies in the entire system, in which case a local application alone would not be sufficient. The entire body would have to be brought into better functioning. The following cases outline a number of applications which have helped us greatly and should do the same for you if you have similar problems.

CASE No. 1: FOOT PERSPIRATION

As a young man my husband was rather unhappy about his excessive foot perspiration which even frequent washings, as often as three times a day, did not improve. I am certain that if he had walked barefoot frequently as a child and adolescent, a better balance would have been established in his system and he would not have suffered from excessive perspiration. To cure one's self of this unpleasant state, the following applications are necessary:

1. FULL SPONGING:

Once a day during first week, twice a week thereafter as long as needed (for details see Chapter 2, Case No. 1, also Comments).

2. SHORT WRAPPING:

Twice during first week, once a week for three additional weeks, once a month thereafter as long as needed (for details see Chapter 40, also Comments).

3. HALF BATH:

Twice during second week, once a week thereafter (for details see Chapter 6, 3, also Comments).

4. HAY-FLOWER FOOT WRAPPING:

One every other day for two hours during first week, once a week thereafter, as long as needed (for details see Chapter 13, Case No. 2).

5. HAY-FLOWER FOOT BATH:

Once a day during second and third week, once a week thereafter, as long as needed.

SUPPLIES:

1. a large bucket, deep enough for the water to reach over the ankles,
2. one cupful of hay flowers
3. two gallons of boiling water
4. a large bucket filled with the coldest water possible.

PROCEDURE:

1. Pour boiling water over hay flowers in bucket, cover and let steep until water reaches a temperature of 90 to 95°,
2. remove shoes and stockings but otherwise remain fully dressed
3. immerse both feet in the hay-flower bath (strained or unstrained) for ten minutes,
4. remove feet from warm bath and put them immediately into the cold water for half a minute,
5. repeat 3. and 4. twice,
6. without drying, after the cold bath, put on stockings

and shoes, and walk around until feet feel warm and dry—in the house during the cold weather.

Comments on Foot Wrapping

When applying these foot wrappings it will seem to you as if they soaked up all impurities. At the same time you will find them strengthening and healing. They are also very beneficial for aching and swollen feet. They have a good effect on the entire body, including the head, and often improve the hearing.

Comments on Foot Baths

These foot baths complement the wrappings, particularly in the strengthening of the feet. They are beneficial for open wounds, swellings, swollen joints, cartilage, infected nails.

GENERAL

All in all, these various applications will bring a good balance into your "total body" system and thereby not only improve your general health but regulate the rate of perspiration factors so that you will never again be bothered with the unpleasantness of excessive foot perspiration.

CASE No. 2: EXCESSIVE HEAD PERSPIRATION

In his later years my husband had taken cold-water applications only very rarely, since he did not feel any need for them. However, when he found that his head perspiration became excessive when he did strenuous work or exercise, he took the following applications:

1. HALF BATH:

Twice during first week, once a week thereafter (for details see Chapter 6, 3, also Comments).

2A. UPPER SPRAY:

Twice during first week, one a week thereafter (for details see Chapter 11, 1, also Comments). Or

2B. UPPER SPONGING:

Twice during first week, once a week thereafter until ready for upper spray (for details see Chapter 8, Case No. 1, 3, also Comments).

Comments

These applications stimulate better activity throughout your whole system and balance not only the natural warmth of your body but also the entire perspiration rate, bringing it to a more normal functioning. If you feel that your perspiration should be brought into proper balance, try applying these treatments conscientiously. You will find that you will derive immediate benefits, and that the body will automatically function at your best normal rate of perspiration.

CASE No. 3: EXCESSIVE NIGHT PERSPIRATION

If you ever wake up during the night finding yourself bathed in perspiration—a sign that your entire system is weak and needs building up—you may want to make the following applications:

1. FULL SPONGING:

One every day during first week, or as often as you wake up during the night, one every other day during second week, once a week thereafter (for details see Chapter 2, Case No. 1, also Comments).

2. SHORT WRAPPING (COLD):

Twice during first week, once a week for 3 weeks thereafter (for details see Chapter 40, also Comments).

Comments

If you put these applications to the test you will find, as I did, that gradually you regain your strength and your perspiration is normalized. Although the progress may be slow at times, you will enjoy constant improvement.

CASE No. 4: EXCESSIVE PERSPIRATION AT MODERATE EXERCISE

If you find yourself perspiring easily at the slightest physical activity, which happens quite often after a more serious illness, then your whole system is still weak. Following is a program to control this type of excessive perspiration:

1. FULL SPONGING:

One every day during first week, or as often as you are wet from perspiration, one every other day during second week, one a week during three weeks thereafter (for details see Chapter 2, Case No. 1, also Comments). Or

2. FULL BATHS:

As often as the Full Sponging (for details see Chapter 10,4, also Comments).

Comments

Whenever I became "soaking wet" from perspiration while doing moderate work, I undressed quickly and sponged myself with cold water as outlined in Chapter 2, Case No. 1, and either went straight to bed or put on dry clothes as quickly as possible (without drying myself), keeping moderately active for about fifteen minutes until I was dry (outside if the weather was warm, otherwise in a warm room).

Later I found that the cold full bath improved my condition much faster. Therefore I kept a tub filled with cold water so that if I perspired during moderate work, I could go right into the tub (as outlined in Chapter 10,4) and otherwise proceed the same as after a full sponging. After two weeks my entire system was in a much better shape. If you apply these spongings or baths you will feel much stronger soon afterward and have a zest for beneficial moderate exercise to utilize your new-found energy.

36

Help for Stomach Ulcers and Heartburn

There have been no stomach ulcers in our family; neither do we suffer from heartburn. But we have always eaten well-balanced and regular meals, on time, not too hot or too spicy, not too rich or too much, not too fast, etc. In addition, we have taken cold-water applications more or less regularly as a general health builder, and our physical and nervous systems, including the stomach, are in a strong and healthy condition. However, if your stomach needs any special attention, the applications indicated in the next two cases may serve you as a guide.

CASE No. 1: STOMACH ULCERS

A friend of mine has been suffering from stomach ulcers for a number of years and has also been under the care of a number of physicians, without any cure ever being achieved. When she heard about the cold-water applications I took for various ailments, she asked me what I would do if I had stomach ulcers. Here are the applications I suggested to her:

1. FULL SPONGING WITH VINEGAR-WATER:

One every evening for two weeks (for details see Chapter 2, Case No. 1) with the following change under

SUPPLIES:

> 2. a basin filled with half vinegar and half cold water (if a rash develops, use less vinegar),

2. HAY-FLOWER COMPRESS ON ABDOMEN:

One every day for two weeks, one every other day during third week, twice a week during fourth week, once a week during fifth week (for details see Chapter 8, Case No. 1, 4 and Comments).

3. TWO HERBS TEA:

One cupful daily, taken one-third morning, noon, and night, for five weeks

PREPARATION:

Boil slowly for ten minutes one teaspoonful of scouring rush and ten crushed juniper berries in one cupful of water, strain.

4. SAUERKRAUT JUICE (WITHOUT CHEMICAL PRESERVATIVES):

Daily one tablespoonful every hour for eight hours during five weeks.

PREPARATION:

Mix one tablespoonful of sauerkraut juice with seven tablespoonfuls of plain water.

5. MILK DIET:

As may be prescribed by doctor.

6. HIP SPRAY:

Once a day during third week, one every other day during fourth and fifth week, once a week thereafter (for details see Chapter 7, Case No. 1, 1, also Comments).

7. UPPER SPRAY:

One a day during third week, one every other day during fourth and fifth week, once every two weeks thereafter (for details see Chapter 11, 1, also Comments).

Comments

My friend has used the foregoing applications alternately with beneficial results whenever she found time, but could not keep them up regularly. If she is in pain, she applies the hay-flower compress to get relief. However, the compress alone will not heal ulcers, but the whole body and its nervous system has to be brought into balance by the various applications.

If you have any sign of stomach ulcers you probably want to use these applications immediately, before the ulcers become very painful. You will find that these applications strengthen and tone your entire system and make you feel glad.

CASE No. 2: HEARTBURN

If I ever suffered from heartburn, I should want to do something that would be of lasting benefit, and I am sure you feel the same way about it. Try the following applications:

1. SPONGING OF ABDOMEN:

Once every morning and evening during first week.

PROVISIONS:

1. ,a small bowl of half cold water and half vinegar put in front of your bed (if rash develops use less vinegar the next time).
2. a facecloth and dry towel,

PROCEDURE:

1. wash entire abdomen thoroughly in even strokes
2. without drying cover lightly with dry towel,
3. cover up with bedding and stay in bed for at least one-half hour.

2. FULL SPONGING:

One every other day during second week, one a week thereafter as long as needed (for details see Chapter 2, Case No. 1, also Comments).

3. VINEGAR-WATER COMPRESS:

One every other day during second week (alternating with full sponging), one a week for two weeks thereafter (for details see Chapter 17, Case No. 1, also Comments).

4. HALF BATH:

One every other day during third week, one a week regularly thereafter (for details see Chapter 6, 3, also Comments).

5. THREE-HERBS TEA MIXTURE:

One tablespoonful every hour for eight hours during first three days, one cupful daily, thereafter taken one-third morning, noon, and night, as long as needed (for details see Chapter 39, 5, also Comments).

Comments on 1. Sponging of Abdomen

This increases beneficial internal warmth throughout the body, giving it strength at the same time, and brings better activity not only in the stomach and intestines but in the entire sysem.

You will find comments on the other applications under the various chapters as indicated.

37

Strengthening Nerves

The regular use of cold-water applications has definitely also affected the functioning nervous systems advantageously in our family. If there was ever any need for the strengthening of our nerves, the following applications would have been applied by us (they can be used even by a beginner):

1. WALKING ON WET STONES OR IN WATER:

Twice daily during first and second week, once daily during third week (for details see Chapter 13, Case No. 1, 1, also Comments).

2. UPPER SPONGING:

Twice daily (morning and evening) during second week, once daily during third week (for details see Chapter 8, Case No. 1, 3, also Comments).

3. KNEE SPRAY:

Once daily during third and fourth week, three times a week regularly thereafter (for details see Chapter 11, 2, also Comments).

4. UPPER SPRAY:

One a day during fourth and fifth week (mornings), twice a week thereafter as long as needed (for details see Chapter 11, 1, also Comments).

5. SITZ BATH:

One every other evening during fourth week (for details see Chapter 9, 2, also Comments).

6. HALF BATH:

One every afternoon during fifth week, once a week regularly thereafter (for details see Chapter 6, 3, also Comments).

7. BACK SPRAY:

One every other morning during sixth week, once a week thereafter as long as needed (for details see Chapter 12, 3, also Comments).

Comments

It may take a while before you feel the benefits of these applications. However, slight indications should already be evident after the first week, with ever-increasing signs of strength in body and mind and of sounder sleep. Courage and joy will return, and you will feel fresh and healthy again.

It is very beneficial to combine these applications with work in the garden or a daily walk in the park of at least a mile, which should take about half an hour.

38

How I Improved Blurred Vision

After we had moved to the country I noticed one summer that my eyes were watering and I assumed that I had developed a slight allergy, which I expected to stop in the fall. Therefore I did not pay any attention to it, and in the fall my eyes were normal again. This was repeated in ensuing summers, but in addition my right eye looked inflamed on certain days. Once in a while my vision became blurred and I had to dry my eyes to be able to see normally again. However, one day I noticed that although my eyes were dry, the vision on my right eye was still blurred and that I had a red spot on the right side of the cornea. You will realize that I was quite alarmed and could not understand what had caused the blur. It was then that I had to do something about my eye with water.

Because I use cold-water applications for my entire system regularly and therefore enjoy very good health, I assumed that the condition of my eye was a local one brought about by allergy and therefore did not plan any general applications such as hip, back, and full spray, but used the following purely local applications:

1. EYE BATH:

One every morning for four weeks (Figure 27 following shows you how to proceed) for which I arranged the following

SUPPLIES:

1. a medium-size bowl with cold water
2. a dry towel, and followed this

PROCEDURE:

1. I dipped my eyes and forehead into the bowl,
2. opened my eyes in the water for about five seconds,
3. took my head out of the water and blinked my eyes for about half a minute,
4. repeated 1. to 3. four times,
5. dried my eyes and face.

2. HONEY:

One drop in the eye every day one hour after eye bath for four weeks.

3. ALUM-WATER EYE RINSE:

Twice a day, afternoon and evening, every three days, alternating with 4. and 5. for four weeks,

PREPARATION:

one-eighth teaspoonful of alum powder, dissolved in one-half cupful of water (lukewarm or cold).

PROCEDURE:

I filled an eyeglass (eyecup) with alum water and rinsed the eye two or three times. You may also apply a piece of gauze dipped in the alum water and wash out the eye carefully.

4. ALOE-WATER EYE RINSE:

Twice a day, afternoon and evening, every three days, alternating with 3. and 5. for four weeks.

PREPARATION:

To one-eighth teaspoonful of aloe powder add one-half cupful of boiling water, stir and let steep for five minutes, cool.

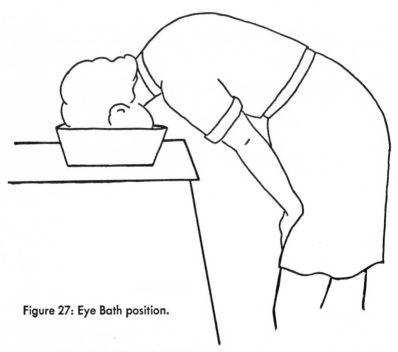

Figure 27: Eye Bath position.

5. WORMWOOD-TEA EYE RINSE:

Twice a day, afternoon and evening, every three days, alternating with 3. and 4. for four weeks.

PREPARATION:

To one-eighth teaspoonful of wormwood add one-half cupful of boiling water, let steep for five minutes and cool, strain.

6. POT-CHEESE EYE COMPRESS:

One every other day during fifth week alternating with 7.

PROCEDURE:

For details see Chapter 41 under POT CHEESE.

7. SCOURING-RUSH EYE COMPRESS:

One every other day during fifth week alternating with 6.

SUPPLIES:

1. a small handkerchief folded twice (into four layers)
2. a hand towel
3. scouring-rush tea, prepared by boiling one teaspoonful of scouring rush in one cupful of water slowly for about five minutes and straining it.

PROCEDURE:

(For details see Chapter 5, Case No. 2, 1.)

8. REPETITION:

of 1. to 7. during the ensuing five weeks, or a total of ten weeks.

Comments on Eye Bath

Eye baths are beneficial not only for weak eyes, but for healthy eyes. George Bernard Shaw is reported to have taken a cold eye bath every day. It preserved his eyesight so that he never needed to wear glasses. Healthy eyes are kept strong by the cold eye bath, and weak eyes are strengthened and refreshed. If the eyes are inflamed, then the eye bath should be taken as often as once every hour.

Comments on Honey and Eye Rinses

Honey cleanses, heals, and strengthens the eye. Although the eyes sting and fill with tears at first, it is only for a moment, and soon the honey soothes any pain and the eyes feel quite relieved.

The alum, aloe, and wormwood dissolve impurities and heal the eyes. Aloe also helps to improve the sight. But it should not be used too often or too long (neither should alum).

Comments on Compresses

The pot-cheese compress is soothing and cooling. It takes the heat and fever out of the eye and thereby reduces the inflammation. Also the scouring-rush compress heals and draws out impurities.

I continued the eye rinses and the eye baths until my eye regained its former strength.

39

Help for a Rash

My family has never experienced a rash of any kind because we have taken cold-water applications either regularly or at least from time to time, thereby purifying our entire system and keeping it in good balance. However, should any member of my family ever have a rash, no matter on what part of the body, I should use, or advise the use of, applications on the entire body as follows (they would also be of great benefit to you if you are suffering from a rash):

1. FULL SPONGING:

One every day during first week (for details see Chapter 2, Case No. 1, also Comments).

2. SHORT WRAPPING:

One every Monday and Thursday during second, third and fourth week (for details see Chapter 40, method A or B, also Comments).

3. UPPER SPRAY:

One every Tuesday and Friday during second, third and fourth week (for details see Chapter 11, 1, also Comments).

4. HIP SPRAY:

One every Wednesday and Saturday during second, third and fourth week, one a week thereafter (for details see Chapter 7, Case No. 1, 1, also Comments).

5. THREE-HERBS TEA MIXTURE:

One cupful daily, one-third morning, noon, and night, for four weeks.

SUPPLIES:

1. Half teaspoonful of sage leaves (cut),
2. half teaspoonful of scouring rush,
3. one tiny leaf of wormwood,
4. one cupful of boiling water,

PROCEDURE:

1. Pour boiling water over three herb teas,
2. cover and let steep for ten minutes, strain,
3. drink before meals, one-third cupful morning, noon, and night, warm or cold as desired,
4. if too bitter (from wormwood) add more water, never any sugar.

Comments: General

You may be inclined to keep the rash dry, but you don't have to be afraid that water would do any harm. Even if in the beginning the rash seems to get worse, this would only be a good sign that the applications are effective in cleaning out all impurities. Since the cause for the rash may be deep-seated, it is important to work on the entire system, thereby enabling it to discard all impurities. Applications 2. to 5. should be continued until the rash is completely disappeared. They will benefit the body in many ways and restore health and strength.

It may happen that if applications for other ailments are made, a rash develops where no rash was before. This also would be a good sign that the applications are effective and the body is discharging the impurities through the particular area.

Comments on 2. Short Wrapping

If the rash is widespread, method B would be preferable, since the herb tea would add to the healing process. The duration of the wrapping depends on your physical strength. A wrapping of one-hour duration is advisable for weak persons. If the rash appears on areas which are not covered by the short wrapping, these areas may be washed several times a day with scouring-rush tea.

Comments on 5. Herb Tea

This herb-tea mixture is not only beneficial for liver, kidneys, stomach and intestines, but also helps to cleanse the blood and purify the system, with the final result of a healthy skin. However, the tea alone cannot be of lasting benefit and achieve the desired result. It must be combined with the other applications.

40

The Great Benefits
of a Short Wrapping

Because the short wrapping is of utmost importance and can be applied by anyone, whether sick or well, at any time without additional applications, this chapter is devoted entirely to its application. For your convenience I am repeating its method of procedure. If you want to have the greatest benefits and also like to be sure that there are no negative effects because of faulty application, the outlined method should be followed very closely.

Figure 28 will guide you in the correct application with the help of an assistant,

Figure 29 shows you how you may proceed in its self-application.

METHOD A—WITH COLD WATER:

SUPPLIES:

1. A bedsheet 108 inches long, folded twice (once in length and once in width), resulting in four layers, to reach from under the armpits almost down to the knees,
2. a woolen blanket folded double,
3. a thin plastic sheet to extend about an inch at the top and bottom of the folded blanket.

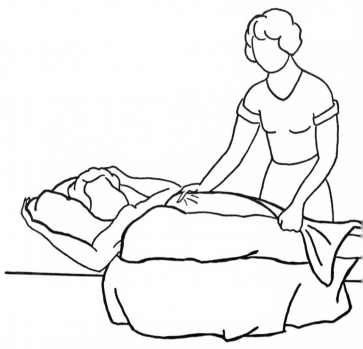

Figure 28: Short Wrapping as applied by another person.

Figure 29: Short Wrapping as self-applied.

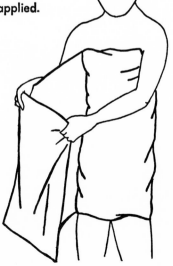

PROCEDURE:

1. The bed is lined with the plastic sheeting,
2. the folded blanket is placed on top of the plastic sheet,
3. the folded bedsheet is dipped into cold water, wrung out carefully (not too dry, but not dripping wet) and spread on the blanket, with the latter extending about an inch on the top and the bottom,
4. you place yourself—completely undressed—on the wet sheet in such a way that the upper edge reaches to the armpits.
5. the sides of the wet sheet are folded over to cling closely to the body, first the one side and then the other, overlapping each other and closing well on top and bottom so that no air can enter,
6. the sides of the blanket are folded over in the same manner, again closing well on the top and bottom, but not too tight,
7. a pajama top and cardigan are pulled over the arms, backside in front, and tucked in on the sides so that the arms may be kept out if desired,
8. the regular bed covers are placed up to the armpits, or up to the chin if preferred, and tucked in all around, especially under the shoulder blades,
9. after one hour remove entire wrapping without drying, put on pajamas and stay well covered in bed for about forty minutes to feel comfortably warm, and dry. For better results the short wrapping should be applied for one and a half hours, however not without dipping the sheet again in cold water after the first forty-five minutes. Since it is difficult to do this alone without being exposed too long, it is not advisable to try it without the help of another person. One should stay under the covers as much as possible. The wet sheet can be pulled from under the body and can be replaced while one rolls over to the far edge of the bed, but always under the covers. The procedures 4. to 9. are then to be repeated.

METHOD B—WITH WARM HERB-TEA WATER OF EITHER HAY FLOWERS, SCOURING RUSH, OR CAMOMILE, ETC.

SUPPLIES:

1.-3. the same as under Method A,
4. Four heaping tablespoonfuls of herbs in a large bucket or bowl with four quarts of boiling water added, letting it steep for about ten minutes.

PROCEDURE:

1.-2. the same as under Method A,
3. the folded bedsheet is dipped into the warm, unstrained herb tea, wrung out carefully, etc. the same as under Method A,
4. to 9. the same as under Method A.
   For better results the warm wrapping also should be applied for one and a half hours, however, not without dipping the sheet again after forty-five minutes, this time into the cold herb tea. For further details and regarding help see under Method A.

Comments

Most of the time the short wrapping should be taken cold. At first you will be freezing for a few minutes, but soon a very agreeable warmth will develop and you will feel pleasantly relaxed. If you take this wrapping regularly, say about once a month, a great number of illnesses can be avoided, because impurities in the body are drawn out through the pores into the wrapping. When removing the white sheet afterward you will find that it has become yellowish in color, or when rinsing it that the water is gray and cloudy. This will prove to you the good effect of the wrapping. It has a cleansing effect not only on the skin and bones, but on all organs as well, such as liver, heart, kidneys, lungs, stomach, sexual organs etc., also on the intestines and even throat and head.

Elderly and weak persons should start with a warm wrapping for one hour only. This is also advisable for sick persons if they feel chilly. However, when taking a warm wrapping it is best to add herbs to the water as described under Method B, especially for certain types of illnesses, as outlined under these illnesses, because of the herbs' added healing effect.

The short wrapping, in whatever form given, should not get so warm that a person starts perspiring. If this happens, the bedsheet should be dipped again in cold water, since otherwise its effects would be weakening. Its purpose is to soften, dissolve, and to draw out impurities of any nature, which it does quite successfully.

41

A Compilation of Herbs
and Other Natural Healing Agents
and Our Experiences in Using Them

In the previous chapters you will have found that in connection with cold-water applications we frequently also used herbs, steeped in boiling water for five minutes, mostly one teaspoonful to a cup (for bitter teas correspondingly less), used either as beverage or prepared in a warm compress. This chapter will give you these herbs and also other healing agents in alphabetical order with added descriptions. In each case the first paragraph identifies the substance, and the second paragraph gives you our experience in its use.

Some of the herbs grow on our lawn, our walks and other open spaces, but we bought most of them either at the drugstore or health-food store. If they are not available there, you can ask your local drugstore or health-food store to get them for you, or refer you to an herbal supplies distributor. Also, you might consult the listing of distributors of herbals in the book, *NATURE'S MEDICINES: The Folklore, Romance, and Value of Herbal Remedies*, which is published by Parker Publishing Company (1966), West Nyack, N.Y.

ALOE

*It grows chiefly in South Africa and is
used as a purgative, tonic, and also em-
menagogue (used to stimulate menstrual
flow).*

To make a usable solution put half a teaspoonful (less if too
irritating) of powdered aloe into a glass or cup, add three-fourths of
a cup of boiling water and let it steep for about five minutes after
which it is ready for use. As an eye rinse three or four times a day,
it is beneficial for watery eyes and cloudy vision. It helps clearing
and healing the eyes. It also heals open wounds very quickly,
whether they are new or old, even if they are deep and filled with
pus. A piece of gauze is dipped into the aloe water and put on the
wound.

ALUM

*Often called common alum or ordinary
alum, used internally as an emetic and
locally as an astringent and styptic.*

Alum has helped us greatly as a mouth rinse for bleeding gums,
or as a gargle for sore throats. We take about half a teaspoonful to
a glass of cold water. For open wounds, the powder can be dusted
on directly. I have even used a very thin solution to wash out my
eye in order to remove cloudiness.

ARNICA

*It grows in the Northern Hemisphere. Its
tincture is used as an embrocation for
bruises, sprains, swellings, etc.*

Our family has been using the tincture on cuts and bruises instead of iodine. The pain usually stopped instantly and the wounds
healed very easily. Gargling with half a cupful of cold water to
which half a teaspoon of arnica tincture has been added helps
clearing the voice.

CAMOMILE

The foliage and flower heads are strong-scented and contain a bitter medicinal principle which is used as an antispas-modic, a diaphoretic, etc.

You will find that this herb is beneficial for feverish colds, cramps, stomach-aches, and congestion if one teaspoonful is steeped in a cup of boiling water for five minutes and then used as a beverage about three times a day.

CHARCOAL

The dictionary merely states that it is used in various processes.

As you probably know, charcoal tablets are often prescribed by doctors. We have found them to assist the digestion and remove gases if taken two or three tablets (the equivalent of a tablespoonful) in a glass of milk. They may also be beneficial for liver ailments.

CENTAURIUM

A genus of herbs, family Gentianaceae. Synonym Erythraea.

This is a very bitter herb. Therefore we usually take only a quarter teaspoonful for each cup of boiling water. More water may be added if it is too bitter, but no sugar. This is very helpful for a stomach-ache and stomach gases, heartburn and digestion in general. We have also taken it to improve liver and kidney functioning.

DANDELION

A well-known plant, abundant as a weed. The herbage is tonic. The root has been used as a diuretic, stomachic and cholagogue.

We eat young dandelion leaves in the spring as a salad, right off our lawn or walks—not because we like it, but because of its cleansing properties, which are excellent not only for the stomach, congested lungs, the lower organs, especially the kidneys, but also for the blood in general and hemorrhoids in particular.

ELDERBERRY

These berries are often made into wine.
They are also diaphoretic and aperient.
This is a very valuable bush of which not only the berry can be used, but also the leaves, blossoms and roots. We drink tea made out of the blossoms because of its cleansing effect on the blood. The berries have the same effect, also on the stomach; they improve urination and health of the kidneys.

FENNEL

A perennial European herb. It is culti-
vated for the aromatic flavor of its seed.
You will find that these seeds are beneficial for colic if one tablespoonful is boiled for five minutes in a cup of milk. It should be taken as warm as possible. If the powder is used as a condiment in food, it gets rid of stomach and intestinal gases. It can also be used as rinsing water for the eyes if one teaspoonful is boiled in a cupful of water for about five minutes.

FENUGREEK (Fenum Graecum, lit. Greek hay)

Annual Asiatic herb with aromatic seeds
used in making curry.
We have found this to be an excellent means of healing boils and open wounds. A little boiling water is added to the powder, which swells considerably and turns into a paste almost like plain peanut butter. It is then spread on a piece of cotton or linen cloth and applied like a plaster on the wound or boil. It even induces swellings to open up by concentrating the impurities into pus in one spot, drawing all unclean matter out gently and closing the wound and healing it only after it is absolutely clean. It soothes and cools, is never painful but extremely effective. The plaster should be renewed every morning and evening. It comes off very easily.

HAY FLOWERS

This word apparently does not exist in the dictionary. It probably is not even the correct word for what it represents, namely the blossoms and seeds left on the barn floor after the hay has been removed, sometimes mixed with short pieces of hay.

We have used the hay flowers mainly for warm compresses, mostly on the abdomen, either for the bladder, kidneys, or other organs. These compresses are also beneficial for rheumatic pains, and arthritis. Warm baths with hay flowers are to be recommended for skin disorders, rashes, boils and open wounds.

HIPROSE (or dog-rose)

It is a common European wild rose.

We drink the split seeds as tea frequently with our meals, instead of the regular tea. For each cup I boil a teaspoonful in water for about five minutes. These seeds have purifying qualities for bladder and kidneys, even if stones and grit are present.

HONEY

A sweet viscid material elaborated in the honey sac of bees out of the nectar of flowers . . . a favorite article of food.

Its healing qualities are not familiar to all. One teaspoonful in a cup of herb tea is beneficial for the stomach and also for colds. One teaspoonful in a glass of water may be used for gargling and also as an eye rinse. By using one drop of honey in my eye every day I have had the most astonishing result which you may read in Chapter 38.

IVY

A well-known climbing or prostrate woody vine with evergreen leaves. . . . In the U.S. is usually called English ivy.

These leaves have served us well for corns on our toes. All that is necessary for you to do is to crush a leaf and tie it over the corn during the night. You will find the corn so soft that single layers can be scraped off with the fingernail. If the corn is hard and thick, this procedure will have to be repeated until finally the entire corn is removed.

JUNIPER

The blue, berrylike fruits of common juni-
per have a warm, pungent taste. The
acrid oil is employed in medicine as a
diuretic and stimulant.

We have found the following procedure beneficial for a weak stomach: Chew four berries the first day, increase one berry a day until fifteen berries are taken, then decrease again one berry a day to four berries. The berries are also helpful for liver and kidney ailments; they clear impurities out of the intestines and improve the blood.

KNOTGRASS

The common cosmopolitan weed (Polyg-
onum aviculare) having jointed stems.

This herb has been used for congestion of lungs, stomach ulcers and bleeding, also for kidneys and stones. It should be taken one small cup morning, noon and night, daily.

LINDENS

Lindens are trees of fine proportions with
large cordate leaves and cymose yellow-
ish flowers which abound in honey.

We have been drinking tea made of the blossoms because of its cleansing properties for kidneys and lungs.

MELON SEEDS (German Kuerbiskerne)

Melons are in the gourd family, the cu-
curbitaceae.

I assume the German Kuerbis is also in that family. However, since I did not know the corresponding type of melon in this country, I ordered the "Kuerbiskerne" from Goodman Pharmacy, 1614 Second Avenue, New York, N.Y. 10028. To get rid of a tapeworm, my family has found the following effective.

PREPARATION:

1. I chopped four ounces of seeds as fine as possible,
2. added enough water to cover them,
3. boiled them over a very low flame for ten minutes.

PROCEDURE:

1. For supper the night before, drink only liquids.
2. Instead of breakfast the following morning eat the four ounces of boiled seeds together with the water —and nothing else.
3. At lunch, have the usual regular meal.

Late the following evening the entire tapeworm was discarded.

NETTLE

These are coarse herbs armed with sting-
ing hairs.

We have included these in our herb teas because they cleanse the blood and kidneys. In Europe they are also eaten as a vegetable like spinach.

PLANTAIN

A large genus of short-stemmed herbs,
being among the commonest weeds. They
are chiefly dooryard or roadside weeds
with narrow or elliptic leaves and spikes
of minute greenish flowers.

These herbs grow plentifully on our lawn and walks. It is good to gather these leaves, crush out the juice and drink it. It purifies the blood. It also heals fresh wounds. If sufficient juice cannot be pressed out, then the leaf itself should be put on the wound. The dried leaves prepared as tea are good to clear congestions.

PEPPERMINT

A pungent and aromatic mint with dark-
green lanceolate leaves.

We have successfully used peppermint tea for nausea, vomiting, improper digestion, especially when in a weakened condition. One cup every morning and evening improves digestion.

PIMPINELLA

A large genus of herbs of the carrot family. (The garden species is anise.)

This tea has been found to be excellent for congestion, especially if a teaspoonful of honey is added to a cup of tea, cleaning lungs and stomach, even kidney and bladder stones, and being beneficial for arthritis.

POT CHEESE

The drained curd of soured milk.

Pot cheese should be used in its original state and not when creamed, as for instance in creamed cottage cheese. It is to be pressed through a fine strainer and stirred to a soft, smooth consistency, for which purpose a few drops of cold water or skimmed milk are added. If you make your own pot cheese, then it is best to add the water which separated from the milk during the process of making the cheese. The prepared pot cheese is ready for use if it can be spread like soft peanut butter or like a salve.

As you probably know, pot cheese is the standing diet for stomach ulcers. However, it is more beneficial as a healing agent if taken frequently during the day in small quantities, either a tablespoonful five or six times a day or, what is even better, a teaspoonful every hour.

When applied externally a pot-cheese poultice works wonders for a great number of inflammations, whether they are external or internal, even on the eyes. The prepared pot cheese should be spread on a piece of cotton or linen, placed on the inflammation and covered with a dry towel, folded into two or four layers. It is to be renewed as soon as it becomes dry, after about fifteen or twenty minutes each, and should be applied for at least an hour. After complete removal, cover with dry towel for half an hour. Burning and stinging pains are reduced immediately, not only of open wounds but also of interior inflammations. It is amazing how this poultice not only takes the heat out of the inflammation but apparently also draws all impurities out through the pores.

POTENTILLA ANSERINA

A large genus of herbs abundant in temperate regions.

We have found the tea made out of this herb to be excellent for various cases of cramps, whether in the chest, the abdomen, the head, or the legs, etc. You may apply it externally by putting very hot compresses of a strong tea solution on the afflicted parts. However it is best to drink the tea strong and very hot as often as necessary, even steeped in boiling milk for about five minutes.

SAGE LEAVES

(Middle English sauge, from Latin salvia, fr. salvus "well" in allusion to its reputed healing virtues). A half-shrubby mint (Salvia officinalis) with grayish-green, pungent and aromatic leaves which are used in flavoring meats, etc. and as a mild tonic and astringent.

We drink this tea frequently because we like its flavor and also know that it is of benefit to liver, kidneys and stomach, eases congestion and loosens the mucus. It is excellent for gargling and as a compress it cleanses and heals infected wounds.

SCOURING RUSH

The common horsetail (Equisetum hyemale) used, especially in Europe, as a scouring material.

We have found this to be a very valuable herb, not only for nosebleeds, but also bleeding in general, hemorrhages, boils, infected wounds, etc. It cleanses and heals stomach, kidneys and wounds with pus accumulation, eases urination, especially if used in a local steambath.

I like to add here what may be amusing to you, namely the experience I had with our cat. When I found that he was unable to urinate, and if at all then in very small quantities, often mixed with blood, I added to his milk up to 50 per cent of scouring-rush tea which he drank, since it is almost tasteless, all during the day until he had consumed an entire cup of tea in his milk. I repeated this procedure for three days. On the fourth day his urination was normal again. To prevent recurrence I add a little tea to his milk from time to time.

VALERIAN

A drug consisting of the dried roots of the common valerian used as a carminative and calmative, especially in nervous affections.

We have experienced its calming effect on the nerves, for a nervous stomach and nervous heart, as well as for colics.

VIOLET

The plant or its flowers are used in pharmacy and confections.

It is helpful for coughs, headache, gases. Best results are obtained if a cupful of boiling water is poured over a tablespoonful of the herb, letting it steep for about five minutes, and taken two tablespoonfuls every two hours.

WATER CRESS

The pungent leaves are used for salad and as an antiscorbutic.

We eat this herb frequently as a salad or plain with our sandwiches. It cleanses the blood and is beneficial for the stomach and lungs.

WORMWOOD

A European woody herb (Artemisia absinthium) of a bitter, slightly aromatic taste, formerly used as a tonic, but now chiefly in making absinthe.

Since this herb is very bitter, we take only the tiniest leaf to make a cup of tea, mostly in combination with other herbs. It is excellent for the stomach, against nausea, also good for the liver and improves the blood. I have used it for infected eyes as an eye wash with very good results.

YARROW

A strong-scented Eurasian herb (Achillea millefolium), naturalized in North America.

We have found this herb to be beneficial for liver, kidneys, bladder, stomach and intestines if taken as a beverage one-third cupful three times a day.

42

Conclusion

Water has been a real blessing to our family, and I often take a moment of meditation to bless it in gratefulness. It is the symbol of life to me, and I hope and wish that it will be a blessing to many.

In contemplating the nature of water I feel that it is the mother, the life of all material manifestation. It is the most flexible and yet the most solid, the most destructive but, next to air, the most necessary. About three-fourths of the earth as well as of the human body is water. No matter how much it is mixed with other substances, when we distill it, it is cleansed and purified into clear water again so that we can drink it to our benefit. No matter what we do to, or with, water, it always can be returned to itself. If heated to steam it returns to water after being cooled, if frozen to ice it returns to water after being warmed. If we make coffee out of it, or tea, or change it in any other way from its original state, it always maintains its identity, and it may always be recovered no matter what we do to it. When evaporating, it generates magnetism, a vital force, the benefit of which is reaped by us when not drying ourselves after any of the applications given in this book, but going to bed wet and letting the water evaporate.

Our family, the same as most families, enjoys being on or near water, but water as such is to us much more than a beverage (of

213

which most people drink far too little), or a cleansing agent; it is also a healing force. It has—mostly in its cold state—kept us healthy and well all through the years.

The only time we use hot water is for muscle cramps in the leg. If a cramp occurs, we dip a facecloth or face towel in very hot water, wring it out lightly and hold it in place on the afflicted area. As soon as the facecloth gets cool it is immediately replaced by a second one, also dipped into hot water, and the whole procedure is constantly repeated until the cramp has disappeared.

In using the applications of this book, I strongly feel that in addition to the healing benefits received thereby, it is better to act, do something, and thus keep the mind busy with some positive action, rather than to passively allow it to be impressed by the sickness.

These applications have kept us so well that after the children were out of infancy I never had to call a doctor again. The children had only their physical examinations as required by the various schools, and whether taken in grammar and high school, or in college, they always were of the highest rating.

I have stayed away from my job only twice during the last fifteen years. During that time also the menopause passed by without affecting me in any way, either physically or mentally. It did not make any difference in my life, and I am convinced that the cold-water applications repeated below as well as occasionally one or the other application listed in this book have regulated my system and kept me in excellent health:

> *once a week a half bath or a hip spray,*
> *three to five times a week a knee spray, arm spray, and a face spray,*
> *as often as possible walking barefoot.*

For best results I do not take the same spray every day, but alternate in applications, or skip a day.

I also like to repeat that whenever our children had a temperature or were not feeling well, they actually asked for a cold bath because they knew how good they would feel soon afterward. And I am delighted and pleased that the same also applies to our grandchildren. Whenever they are really sick they say: "Mommy,

I want a cold bath." They know from experience that water is the answer.

I have often heard the remark: "I don't see how water can help." It does! Just try it! You have my experience in proof of what is said in this book.

INDEX